T0227358

Stage B, a Pre-cursor of Heart Failure, Part II

Guest Editors

JAY N. COHN, MD
GARY S. FRANCIS, MD

HEART FAILURE CLINICS

www.heartfailure.theclinics.com

Consulting Editors
RAGAVENDRA R. BALIGA, MD, MBA
JAMES B. YOUNG, MD

Founding Editor
JAGAT NARULA, MD, PhD

April 2012 • Volume 8 • Number 2

SAUNDERS an imprint of ELSEVIER, Inc.

W.B. SAUNDERS COMPANY
A Division of Elsevier Inc.

1600 John F. Kennedy Boulevard • Suite 1800 • Philadelphia, Pennsylvania 19103-2899

http://www.theclinics.com

HEART FAILURE CLINICS Volume 8, Number 2
April 2012 ISSN 1551-7136, ISBN-13: 978-1-4557-3872-4

Editor: Barbara Cohen-Kligerman
Developmental Editor: Teia Stone

Heart Failure Clinics (ISSN 1551-7136) is published quarterly by Elsevier Inc., 360 Park Avenue South, New York, NY 10010-1710. Months of publication are January, April, July, and October. Business and editorial offices: 1600 John F. Kennedy Boulevard, Suite 1800, Philadelphia, PA 19103-2899. Periodicals postage paid at New York, NY, and additional mailing offices. Subscription prices are USD 224.00 per year for US individuals, USD 347.00 per year for US institutions, USD 76.00 per year for US students and residents, USD 268.00 per year for Canadian individuals, USD 398.00 per year for Canadian institutions, USD 285.00 per year for international individuals, USD 398.00 per year for international institutions, and USD 96.00 per year for Canadian and foreign students/residents. To receive student and resident rate, orders must be accompanied by name of affiliated institution, date of term, and the *signature* of program/residency coordinator on institution letterhead. Orders will be billed at individual rate until proof of status is received. Foreign air speed delivery is included in all *Clinics* subscription prices. All prices are subject to change without notice. **POSTMASTER:** Send address changes to *Heart Failure Clinics*, Elsevier Health Sciences Division, Subscription Customer Service, 3251 Riverport Lane, Maryland Heights, MO 63043. **Customer Service: 1-800-654-2452 (US and Canada). From outside of the US and Canada, call 314-447-8871. Fax: 314-447-8029. For print support, e-mail: JournalsCustomerService-usa@elsevier.com. For online support, e-mail: JournalsOnlineSupport-usa@elsevier.com.**

Reprints. For copies of 100 or more of articles in this publication, please contact the Commercial Reprints Department, Elsevier Inc., 360 Park Avenue South, New York, NY 10010-1710. Tel.: 212-633-3812; Fax: 212-462-1935; E-mail: reprints@elsevier.com.

Heart Failure Clinics is covered in *MEDLINE/PubMed (Index Medicus)*.

Cover artwork courtesy of Umberto M. Jezek.

Printed and bound by CPI Group (UK) Ltd, Croydon, CR0 4YY

Transferred to Digital Print 2012

Contributors

CONSULTING EDITORS

RAGAVENDRA R. BALIGA, MD, MBA
Vice Chief and Assistant Division Director, Professor of Medicine, Division of Cardiovascular Medicine, The Ohio State University Medical Center, Columbus, Ohio

JAMES B. YOUNG, MD
Professor of Medicine and Executive Dean, Cleveland Clinic Lerner College of Medicine; George and Linda Kaufman Chair, Chairman, Endocrinology and Metabolism Institute, Cleveland Clinic, Cleveland, Ohio

GUEST EDITORS

JAY N. COHN, MD, FACC
Professor of Medicine, Cardiovascular Division, University of Minnesota Medical School, Minneapolis, Minnesota

GARY S. FRANCIS, MD
Professor of Medicine, Division of Cardiovascular Disease, University of Minnesota Medical School, Minneapolis, Minnesota

AUTHORS

INDER S. ANAND, MD, FRCP, DPhil (Oxon), FACC
Professor of Medicine, Department of Medicine, University of Minnesota Medical School; Director, Heart Failure Program, Minneapolis Veterans Affairs Health Care System, Minneapolis, Minnesota

JOHN J. ATHERTON, MBBS, PhD, FRACP, FCSANZ
Director of Cardiology, Department of Cardiology, Royal Brisbane and Women's Hospital, Herston; Associate Professor, University of Queensland School of Medicine, Brisbane, Queensland, Australia

GEORGE A. BELLER, MD
Ruth C. Heede Professor of Cardiology, Division of Cardiology, University of Virginia Health System, Charlottesville, Virginia

SUSAN CHENG, MD
Instructor in Medicine, Division of Cardiovascular Medicine, Department of Medicine, Brigham and Women's Hospital, Boston, Massachusetts

ERIN E. COGLIANESE, MD
Assistant Professor of Medicine, Division of Cardiology, Loyola University Health System, Maywood, Illinois

PATRICK COLLIER, MB, PhD
Heart Failure Unit, St Vincent's University Hospital, Elm Park, Dublin, Ireland

VIOREL G. FLOREA, MD, PhD, ScD, FACC
Assistant Professor of Medicine, Department of Medicine, University of Minnesota Medical School; Heart Failure Program, Minneapolis Veterans Affairs Health Care System, Minneapolis, Minnesota

GARY S. FRANCIS, MD
Professor of Medicine, Division of Cardiovascular Disease, University of Minnesota Medical School, Minneapolis, Minnesota

RAJESH JANARDHANAN, MD, MRCP
Advanced Cardiovascular Imaging Fellow, Division of Cardiology, University of Virginia Health System, Charlottesville, Virginia

JOÃO A.C. LIMA, MD
Professor of Medicine and Radiology,
Departments of Medicine and Radiology,
Johns Hopkins School of Medicine and Johns
Hopkins Hospital, Baltimore, Maryland

KENNETH M. MCDONALD, MD
Director, Heart Failure Unit, St Vincent's
University Hospital, Elm Park, Dublin, Ireland

SARA L. PARTINGTON, MD
Fellow, Non-Invasive Cardiovascular Imaging
Program, Departments of Medicine and
Radiology, Brigham and Women's Hospital,
Boston, Massachusetts

BERTRAM PITT, MD
Professor of Medicine Emeritus,
Cardiovascular Center, University Hospital,
University of Michigan School of Medicine,
Ann Arbor, Michigan

MARGARET M. REDFIELD, MD
Cardiovascular Division, Mayo Clinic,
Rochester, Minnesota

MOHAMMAD SARRAF, MD
Division of Cardiovascular Disease, University
of Minnesota, Minneapolis, Minnesota

ANNE L. TAYLOR, MD
John Lindenbaum Professor of Medicine at
New York Presbyterian Hospital; Vice Dean
for Academic Affairs, Department of Medicine,
Columbia University College of Physicians
and Surgeons, New York, New York

THOMAS J. WANG, MD
Associate Professor of Medicine, Cardiology
Division, Massachusetts General Hospital,
Harvard Medical School, Boston,
Massachusetts

Contents

Estimates of the prevalence of asymptomatic left ventricular systolic dysfunction (LVSD) vary widely depending on the study sample and definition of LVSD. Subtle reductions in LV systolic or diastolic function are now detectable with newer echocardiographic measures, which can influence estimates of the burden of stage B heart failure (HF). If the definition is broadened to include diastolic filling abnormalities, the estimated prevalence of stage B HF increases dramatically. This article reviews the rationale for echocardiographic screening for stage B HF, describes currently available measures of cardiac structure and function, and assesses the potential role of echocardiography in selected subgroups.

Cardiac magnetic resonance imaging (CMR) can play a key role in the assessment and follow-up of patients with stage B heart failure. CMR currently serves as the reference standard for quantifying right and left ventricular size and ejection fraction. Technical advances have also enabled CMR to provide noninvasive tissue characterization and detailed assessments of myocardial performance. Thus, in addition to standard metrics of cardiac structure and function, CMR offers a variety of tools for determining cause, severity, and estimating the prognosis associated with an asymptomatic cardiomyopathy.

This article discusses currently available radionuclide techniques in the diagnostic and prognostic evaluation of patients with chronic heart failure, with a focus on stage B/asymptomatic left ventricular dysfunction. Radionuclide imaging is promising for such patients because it can simultaneously determine left ventricular function, evaluate for the presence of obstructive coronary disease, determine the extent of viable myocardium, and evaluate dyssynchronous left ventricular contraction. Radionuclide imaging can thus provide important noninvasive insights into the pathophysiology, prognosis, and management of patients with asymptomatic left ventricular dysfunction as well as more advanced heat failure.

Epidemiologic, clinical, and basic research has identified several antecedent conditions that predispose individuals to heart failure and its predecessor, asymptomatic left ventricular remodeling and dysfunction (stage B heart failure). Many biochemical markers have been described that characterize the remodeling process and the development of cardiac dysfunction. Although natriuretic peptides and cardiac troponin are currently used in the context of diagnosis, risk stratification, and management of stage C and D heart failure, many other biomarkers provide insights into the underlying pathophysiology of left ventricular dysfunction, suggesting new directions for fundamental research or the development of new therapies.

This article outlines the link between the renin angiotensin aldosterone system (RAAS) and various forms of cardiomyopathy, and also reviews the understanding of the effectiveness of RAAS intervention in this phase of ventricular dysfunction. The authors focus their discussion predominantly on patients who have had previous myocardial infarction or those who have left ventricular hypertrophy and also briefly discuss the role of RAAS activation and intervention in patients with alcoholic cardiomyopathy.

β-blockers are an important treatment of heart failure (HF) and are useful in reducing the progression of the syndrome. They should be considered for patients with asymptomatic left ventricular (LV) dysfunction. Evidence-based β-blocker therapy (bisoprolol, carvedilol, or metoprolol succinate) in combination with standard therapy is a mainstay of treatment of all symptomatic patients with LV systolic dysfunction. Patients in stage B also benefit from the early introduction of β-blockers, but there are no large randomized clinical trials to support this strategy. Whether there is a role for ivabradine in the treatment of HF is not clear.

This article focuses on the potential role of mineralocorticoid receptor antagonists (MRAs) in patients with stage B heart failure (HF) due to hypertension, diabetes mellitus, and/or visceral obesity with the metabolic syndrome. It briefly discusses the role of MRAs in patients with left ventricular dilatation due to nonischemic or ischemic cardiomyopathy and in those with a prior myocardial infarction but without left ventricular dilatation or evidence of HF.

Nitric oxide (NO) is recognized as one of the most important cardiovascular signaling molecules, with multiple regulatory effects on myocardial and vascular tissue as well as on other tissues and organ systems. With the growth in understanding of the range and mechanisms of NO effects on the cardiovascular system, it is now possible to consider pharmaceutical interventions that directly target NO or key steps in NO effector pathways. This article reviews aspects of the cardiovascular effects of NO, abnormalities in NO regulation in heart failure, and clinical trials of drugs that target specific aspects of NO signaling pathways.

To adequately address the burden imposed by heart failure, a combined approach to prevention, early detection, and management is required. Failure to adequately consider the presymptomatic pool of subjects largely accounts for the continuing burden of incident cases of symptomatic heart failure. This article reviews the rationale for the early detection and management of stage B heart failure with specific reference to asymptomatic left ventricular systolic dysfunction as a potentially modifiable heart failure antecedent. Provided one can safely and reliably detect these individuals, a strong case can be made for screening given the evidence from treatment efficacy studies that clinicians can improve patient outcomes.

Heart failure (HF) prevention is an indisputably laudable goal, albeit with undefined global public health impact in an increasingly elderly population with competing cardiovascular and noncardiovascular risks for morbidity and mortality. The understanding of cardiac and noncardiac structural and functional abnormalities that predispose to the diverse clinical HF syndrome is rapidly advancing, and novel approaches for prevention and treatment are needed. Successful approaches mandate not only identification of discrete therapeutic targets but also research into the developing sciences of health care delivery and behavioral modification. Targeting Stage B HF represents one such potential strategy.

Heart Failure Clinics

ACCESS THE CLINICS ONLINE!

Available at:
http://www.theclinics.com

Editorial

Reducing the Burden of Stage B Heart Failure and the Global Pandemic of Cardiovascular Disease: Time to Go to War with the "Barefoot" Troops!

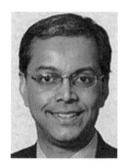
Ragavendra R. Baliga, MD, MBA

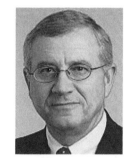
James B. Young, MD

Consulting Editors

Patients with stage B heart failure have structural heart disease but no symptoms of heart failure (HF). Some examples of how asymptomatic (at least from the HF standpoint) systolic and diastolic left ventricular dysfunction can happen include patients having a myocardial infarction, those with left ventricular hypertrophy and low ejection fraction (secondary to hypertension), and those with asymptomatic valvular disease.[1,2] The etiology of stage B heart failure[1,2] is the same as etiology of any stage of HF and includes atherosclerotic heart disease, hypertension, dyslipidemia, obesity, diabetes,[3] metabolic syndrome, cardiotoxins,[4] and rheumatic or other valvular heart disease (**Fig. 1**).[5] Since myocardial infarction and hypertension together account for about three-fourths of the population-attributable risk of HF,[6] and both are preventable with currently available therapies (**Fig. 2**), we have a battlefield target.[7]

In 2008, the Global Burden of Metabolic Risk Factors of Chronic Diseases Collaborating Group reported that 1.46 billion adults were overweight (body mass index [BMI] $\geq$25 kg/m^2), including 500 million who were obese (BMI $\geq$30 kg/m^2); that is, worldwide, one in three adults is overweight and one in nine adults is obese.[8] The

increase in obesity is of concern because obesity has been shown to be a proximate risk factor for HF[9] in the Framingham heart study[10] and may exert its influence both directly and indirectly, by promoting hypertension, diabetes, dyslipidemia, metabolic syndrome, and atherosclerosis. The same Chronic Diseases Collaborating Group reported that 1 billion individuals had uncontrolled hypertension (systolic blood pressure [SBP] $\geq$140 or diastolic [DBP] $\geq$90 mm Hg).[11] This is also of concern because there is a twofold increase in risk of HF among those who have SBP >160 mm Hg and DBP levels >90 mm Hg compared with those who have SBP levels <140 mm Hg and DBP levels <90 mm Hg. This risk is said to be continuous, so HF can be expected among those who have SBP levels >120 mm Hg, although at a lower rate. The increase in obesity, hypertension, dyslipidemia,[12] and smoking in economically growing low-income and middle-income countries is projected to add to the burden of cardiovascular disease in high-income nations and result in a worldwide cardiovascular disease pandemic. The investigators of this collaborating group also found that, despite the increase in obesity, there has been a decline in three factors, namely hypertension, dyslipidemia, and smoking

heartfailure.theclinics.com

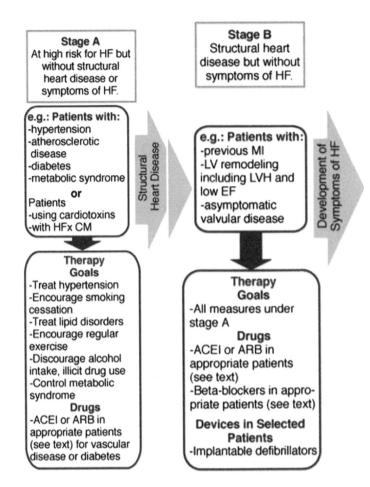

Fig. 1. Stage A and stage heart failure: overview. (*Adapted from* Hunt SA, Abraham WT, Chin MH, et al. ACC/AHA 2005 Guideline Update for the Diagnosis and Management of Chronic Heart Failure in the Adult: a report of the American College of Cardiology/American Heart Association Task Force on Practice Guidelines (Writing Committee to Update the 2001 Guidelines for the Evaluation and Management of Heart Failure): developed in collaboration with the American College of Chest Physicians and the International Society for Heart and Lung Transplantation: endorsed by the Heart Rhythm Society. Circulation 2005;112(12):e154–235; with permission.)

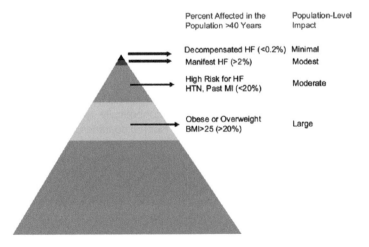

Fig. 2. Pyramid of HF in population. (*From* Young JB, Narula J. Prevention should take center stage. Cardiol Clin 2007;25(4):xi–xiii; with permission.)

cessation, due to therapy in high-income countries, suggesting that targeting these three factors should reduce the burden of cardiovascular disease including HF even though the burden of obesity continues to increase (**Fig. 3**).[13]

A 5-mm Hg drop in a population's SBP is expected to reduce the age-specific rates of HF by about one-fourth. In persons who have hypertension (prevalence, ~20%), a 10-mm Hg reduction in SBP has been shown to reduce the incidence of HF by 50%, even among elderly patients.[14]

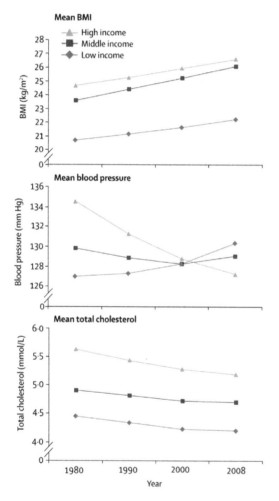

Fig. 3. Change over time in mean BMI, systolic blood pressure, and total cholesterol by countries' income category: BMI is increasing in all three economic categories. In high-income countries, blood pressure and total cholesterol are decreasing. In middle-income countries, there is no major change in blood pressure and total cholesterol is decreasing. In low-income countries, blood pressure is increasing and total cholesterol is decreasing.[13] (*From* Anand SS, Yusuf S. Stemming the global tsunami of cardiovascular disease. Lancet 2011;377(9765):530. [www.thelancet.com]; with permission.)

Pharmacotherapy with lifestyle modifications to lower the mean blood pressure is projected to reduce age-specific rates of HF in the population by more than one-third and possibly by as much as one-half. Statins reduce the incidence of HF by approximately 20% among patients who have dyslipidemia and coronary artery disease.[15] Angiotensin converting enzyme (ACE) inhibitors reduce incidence of HF by 37% among patients who have reduced left ventricular systolic function and by 23% among patients who have coronary artery disease and normal systolic function.[15] Observational studies have reported a lower incidence of HF among diabetics who have better glycemic control.[15]

Despite the known benefits of therapy, all of these effective treatments are underutilized, and control of hypertension is particularly dismal. The Prospective Urban Rural Epidemiological (PURE) study investigators found that very few individuals with cardiovascular disease received statins (14.6%), β-blockers (17.4%), ACE inhibitors or angiotensin receptor blocker (ARBs) (19.5%), or antiplatelet drugs (25.3%). Utilization was lowest in low-income countries (statins, 3.3%; β-blockers, 9.7%; ACE inhibitors or ARBs, 5.2%; and antiplatelet drugs, 8.8%) and greatest in high-income countries (66.5%, 40%, 49.8%, and 62%, respectively), and decreased in line with reduction of country economic status (P_{trend} <.0001 for every drug type).[16] Fewer patients received no drugs in high-income countries (11.2%), compared with 45.1% in upper-middle income countries, 69.3% in lower-middle income countries, and 80.2% in low-income countries. Drug utilization was greater in urban than rural areas (antiplatelet drugs 28.7% urban vs 21.3% rural, β-blockers 23.5% vs 15.6%, ACE inhibitors or ARBs 22.8% vs 15.5%, and statins 19.9% vs 11.6%; all P<.0001), with most variation in low-income countries ($P_{interaction}$ <.0001 for urban vs rural differences by country economic status). In high-income countries, less than 50% of patients get any of these medications after myocardial infarction or stroke; in middle-income countries, 25%–30% of patients get the medications, and in low-income countries less than 10% of individuals get any of these medications (**Fig. 4**). This suggests that about 50% of the patients in high-income countries are getting the same level of care as the poorest countries!

There is a huge opportunity to stamp out the scourge of cardiovascular disease in all countries and this will require an approach similar to that used in China to reduce the burden of "big-belly," the peasant name for schistosomiasis. China successfully utilized physician extenders or *bare-foot doctors* to reduce the burden of polio,

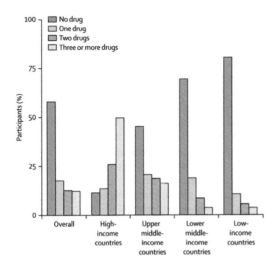

Fig. 4. Number of drugs taken by patients with coronary artery disease by country economic status. The drugs counted were aspirin, β-blockers, ACE inhibitors or ARBs, or statins. (*From* Yusuf S, Islam S, Chow CK, et al. Use of secondary prevention drugs for cardiovascular disease in the community in high-income, middle-income, and low-income countries (the PURE Study): a prospective epidemiological survey. Lancet 2011;378(9798):1231–43; with permission.)

smallpox, and schistosomiasis.[17] A typical barefoot doctor in China graduated from secondary school and practiced in the community after training for only 3–6 months at the county or community hospital.[18] These individuals were schooled in anatomy, microbiology, diagnosing disease, birth control, maternal and infant care, acupuncture, and prescribing traditional and Western medicines. These barefoot doctors provided basic health care: first aid, health education, and immunizations against diphtheria, whooping cough, and measles. When confronted with illnesses beyond their training, these barefoot doctors referred patients to physicians. Despite a low level of service in terms of having sophisticated technology or medical instruments, the barefoot doctor program provided timely treatment to the masses while keeping costs low.[17]

In our opinion, the way to reduce the pandemic of atherosclerotic disease and consequent HF is to attack it in a war-like fashion by mobilizing physician extenders such as the barefoot doctors to provide lifelong primary and secondary preventive therapy,[19–21] including tobacco cessation, salt reduction,[22] improved diets and physical activity, reduction in excessive alcohol intake, and increased utilization of essential low-cost medications, namely statins, antiplatelet agents, ACE inhibitors or ARBs, β-blockers, and other blood pressure reducing medications,[14] possibly as

a "poly-pill."[23–25] We realize that this is a radical suggestion for North America but believe utilization of physician extenders to provide preventive therapy would free the physician to focus on providing other more sophisticated secondary, tertiary, or quaternary health care.

To discuss the opportunities of reducing the burden of Stage B heart failure, Drs Jay Cohn and Gary Francis have assembled a panel of international experts with a passion for preventing cardiovascular disease and reducing the overall burden.[26] In our opinion, this would require an international effort involving extension of the current health care delivery systems to incorporate physician extenders such as "barefoot doctors" to prevent cardiovascular disease—it is time to go "barefoot" to stamp out the raging inferno of cardiovascular disease.

Ragavendra R. Baliga, MD, MBA
Division of Cardiovascular Medicine
The Ohio State University Medical Center
Columbus, OH, USA

James B. Young, MD
Lerner College of Medicine and
Endocrinology & Metabolism Institute
Cleveland Clinic
Cleveland, OH, USA

E-mail addresses:
Ragavendra.baliga@osumc.edu (R.R. Baliga)
youngj@ccf.org (J.B. Young)

REFERENCES

1. Hunt SA, Abraham WT, Chin MH, et al. 2009 Focused update incorporated into the ACC/AHA 2005 Guidelines for the Diagnosis and Management of Heart Failure in Adults: A Report of the American College of Cardiology Foundation/American Heart Association Task Force on Practice Guidelines Developed in Collaboration with the International Society for Heart and Lung Transplantation. J Am Coll Cardiol 2009;53(15):e1–90.

2. Hunt SA, Abraham WT, Chin MH, et al. ACC/AHA 2005 Guideline Update for the Diagnosis and Management of Chronic Heart Failure in the Adult: a report of the American College of Cardiology/ American Heart Association Task Force on Practice Guidelines (Writing Committee to Update the 2001 Guidelines for the Evaluation and Management of Heart Failure): developed in collaboration with the American College of Chest Physicians and the International Society for Heart and Lung Transplantation: endorsed by the Heart Rhythm Society. Circulation 2005;112(12):e154–235.

3. Danaei G, Finucane MM, Lu Y, et al. National, regional, and global trends in fasting plasma glucose and diabetes prevalence since 1980: systematic analysis of health examination surveys and epidemiological studies with 370 country-years and 2.7 million participants. Lancet 2011;378(9785):31–40.

4. Baliga RR, Young JB. Early detection and monitoring of vulnerable myocardium in patients receiving chemotherapy: is it time to change tracks? Heart Fail Clin 2011;7(3):xiii–xix.

5. Young JB. The global epidemiology of heart failure. Med Clin North Am 2004;88(5):1135–43, ix.

6. Lloyd-Jones DM, Larson MG, Leip EP, et al. Lifetime risk for developing congestive heart failure: the Framingham Heart Study. Circulation 2002;106(24):3068–72.

7. Yusuf S, Pitt B. A lifetime of prevention: the case of heart failure. Circulation 2002;106(24):2997–8.

8. Finucane MM, Stevens GA, Cowan MJ, et al. National, regional, and global trends in body-mass index since 1980: systematic analysis of health examination surveys and epidemiological studies with 960 country-years and 9.1 million participants. Lancet 2011;377(9765):557–67.

9. Yusuf S, Anand S. Body-mass index, abdominal adiposity, and cardiovascular risk. Lancet 2011;378(9787):226–7 [author reply: 228].

10. Kenchaiah S, Evans JC, Levy D, et al. Obesity and the risk of heart failure. N Engl J Med 2002;347(5):305–13.

11. Danaei G, Finucane MM, Lin JK, et al. National, regional, and global trends in systolic blood pressure since 1980: systematic analysis of health examination surveys and epidemiological studies with 786 country-years and 5.4 million participants. Lancet 2011;377(9765):568–77.

12. Farzadfar F, Finucane MM, Danaei G, et al. National, regional, and global trends in serum total cholesterol since 1980: systematic analysis of health examination surveys and epidemiological studies with 321 country-years and 3.0 million participants. Lancet 2011;377(9765):578–86.

13. Anand SS, Yusuf S. Stemming the global tsunami of cardiovascular disease. Lancet 2011;377(9765):529–32.

14. Baliga RR. Applying hypertension guidelines to reduce the burden of heart failure. Cardiol Clin 2007;25(4):507–22, v–vi.

15. Baker DW. Prevention of heart failure. J Card Fail 2002;8(5):333–46.

16. Yusuf S, Islam S, Chow CK, et al. Use of secondary prevention drugs for cardiovascular disease in the community in high-income, middle-income, and low-income countries (the PURE Study): a prospective epidemiological survey. Lancet 2011;378(9798):1231–43.

17. Farley J. Bilharzia: a history of imperial tropical medicine. Cambridge; New York: Cambridge University Press; 1991.

18. Zhang D, Unschuld PU. China's barefoot doctor: past, present, and future. Lancet 2008;372(9653):1865–7.

19. Schocken DD, Benjamin EJ, Fonarow GC, et al. Prevention of heart failure: a scientific statement from the American Heart Association Councils on Epidemiology and Prevention, Clinical Cardiology, Cardiovascular Nursing, and High Blood Pressure Research; Quality of Care and Outcomes Research Interdisciplinary Working Group; and Functional Genomics and Translational Biology Interdisciplinary Working Group. Circulation 2008;117(19):2544–65.

20. Young JB, Narula J. Prevention should take center stage. Cardiol Clin 2007;25(4):xi–xiii.

21. Frieden TR, Berwick DM. The "Million Hearts" initiative—preventing heart attacks and strokes. N Engl J Med 2011;365(13):e27.

22. Baliga RR, Narula J. Salt never calls itself sweet. Indian J Med Res 2009;129(5):472–7.

23. Francis GS, Young JB. The looming polypharmacy crisis in the management of patients with heart failure. Potential solutions. Cardiol Clin 2001;19(4):541–5.

24. Lonn E, Bosch J, Teo KK, et al. The polypill in the prevention of cardiovascular diseases: key concepts, current status, challenges, and future directions. Circulation 2011;122(20):2078–88.

25. Yusuf S, Pais P, Afzal R, et al. Effects of a polypill (Polycap) on risk factors in middle-aged individuals without cardiovascular disease (TIPS): a phase II, double-blind, randomised trial. Lancet 2009;373(9672):1341–51.

26. Berry JD, Dyer A, Cai X, et al. Lifetime risks of cardiovascular disease. N Engl J Med 2012;366(4):321–9.

Preface
Stage B, A Precursor of Heart Failure, Part II

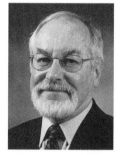
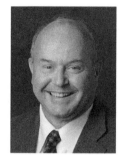

Jay N. Cohn, MD   Gary S. Francis, MD
Guest Editors

This second issue of our series on "Stage B, a precursor of heart failure" deals with the clinical detection and possible management of this pathophysiological process.

The structural abnormalities and the various mechanisms that may contribute to their progression were extensively covered in the first issue. Based on these descriptions, time-dependent worsening of the structural abnormalities and the development of a symptomatic functional abnormality are likely consequences. Thus, clinical assessment to detect and monitor these structural abnormalities and therapeutic approaches to slow or reverse them become a challenge in clinical management.

This issue provides the insights of experts who have long grappled with these problems. Potential monitoring tools are explored in depth, both imaging procedures and biomarker assays. The sensitivity and specificity of these tools are critical in determining their usefulness in the clinical setting.

Neurohormonal inhibiting therapy has served as the cornerstone of treatment for symptomatic patients to inhibit progression of the structural changes. Nitric oxide enhancement appears to provide additional benefit for at least some patients with heart failure. A review of these therapeutic approaches is provided by clinical scientists who have been directly involved in evaluating these agents. How these drugs can or should be used in asymptomatic individuals with structural changes remains largely unexplored. Such trials will be necessary to document efficacy before widespread utilization can be advocated.

Clinical trials in asymptomatic patients with structural abnormalities of the heart will require screening to identify an at-risk population. Much controversy exists on the whole issue of population screening to prevent cardiovascular morbidity and mortality. The rationale for screening and the possible strategies for screening are addressed in the last section of this issue. These are critical issues if we are to move forward in an effort to prevent symptomatic heart failure rather than to deal only with its escalating incidence. An effective strategy to detect and treat these structural precursors of the functional disorder we call "heart failure" could have profound beneficial effects on our exploding health care expenditures.

Jay N. Cohn, MD
Gary S. Francis, MD

University of Minnesota Medical School
Minneapolis, MN 55455, USA

E-mail addresses:
cohnx001@umn.edu (J.N. Cohn)
franc354@umn.edu (G.S. Francis)

doi:10.1016/j.hfc.2012.01.002
1551-7136/12/$ – see front matter © 2012 Elsevier Inc. All rights reserved.

Clinical Monitoring of Stage B Heart Failure: Echocardiography

Erin E. Coglianese, MD[a], Thomas J. Wang, MD[b],*

KEYWORDS

- Stage B heart failure • Heart failure • Echocardiography
- Left ventricular systolic dysfunction

The widespread availability of echocardiography makes it an attractive tool for detecting the structural changes that accompany stage B heart failure (HF). The best studied manifestation of stage B HF is reduced left ventricular ejection fraction (LVEF), or asymptomatic left ventricular systolic dysfunction (LVSD), which is typically assessed echocardiographically. Estimates of the prevalence of asymptomatic LVSD in the community vary widely depending on the study sample and definition of LVSD (**Table 1**).[1] More subtle reductions in left ventricular (LV) systolic or diastolic function are now detectable with newer echocardiographic measures, which can influence estimates of the burden of stage B HF. For instance, if the definition is broadened to include diastolic filling abnormalities, the estimated prevalence of stage B HF increases dramatically.[2]

This article reviews the rationale for echocardiographic screening for screening for stage B HF, describes currently available measures of cardiac structure and function, and assesses the potential role of echocardiography in selected subgroups.

WHY SCREEN FOR LEFT VENTRICULAR SYSTOLIC DYSFUNCTION WITH ECHOCARDIOGRAPHY?

Several investigators have proposed screening programs for LV dysfunction, particularly systolic dysfunction, as a strategy for preventing the onset of overt HF. A critical criterion for screening is the presence of a latent phase of disease whereby an abnormality is present but is not clinically manifest.

Asymptomatic LVSD detected by echocardiography represents such a latent phase in the progression to overt symptomatic HF. Wang and colleagues[3] found a dramatically increased risk of overt HF in individuals with asymptomatic LVSD detected by echocardiography in the Framingham Heart Study. Participants with LVSD in the mild range, defined as an LVEF of 40% to 50%, had a more than threefold risk of developing overt HF compared with those with normal LV function. Individuals with moderate to severe LVSD, defined as LVEF less than 40%, had a nearly eightfold risk. Of importance is that the time to onset of HF in many instances was a decade or more, suggesting a window of opportunity for preventive measures. Further, roughly half of the individuals with LVSD had no prior history of myocardial infarction.[3] As reviewed previously, evidence that early intervention can forestall the development of overt HF is provided by large-scale trials of angiotensin-converting enzyme inhibition, such as the SOLVD Prevention trial.[4] Early intervention in those with diastolic dysfunction, with risk-factor modification and blood-pressure control, may also yield benefits, although data from randomized trials are currently lacking.

ECHOCARDIOGRAPHIC ABNORMALITIES INCLUDED IN THE DEFINITION OF STAGE B HEART FAILURE

The American Heart Association and American College of Cardiology have defined stage B HF as "detectable structural disease without symptoms

[a] Division of Cardiology, Loyola University Health System, 2160 South First Avenue, Maywood, IL 60514, USA
[b] Cardiology Division, Massachusetts General Hospital, Harvard Medical School, Boston, MA, USA
* Corresponding author. Cardiology Division, Massachusetts General Hospital, GRB-800, 55 Fruit Street, Boston, MA 02114.
E-mail address: tjwang@partners.org

Heart Failure Clin 8 (2012) 169–178
doi:10.1016/j.hfc.2011.11.007
1551-7136/12/$ – see front matter © 2012 Published by Elsevier Inc

Table 1
Use of echocardiography to determine prevalence of systolic dysfunction in the population

Study	Participants (n)	Mean Age (y)	Men (%)	Prevalence of Asymptomatic LVSD
LVSD Defined as EF <0.50, or Equivalent				
Strong Heart Study[60]	3184	58	37	12.5
HyperGEN Study[61]	2086	55	38	12.9
Echocardiographic Heart of England Study[62]	3960	61	50	3.3
MONICA project[63]	1566	50	48	1.1
Hedberg et al[64]	412	75	50	3.2
Rotterdam Study[65]	2267	66	45	2.9[a]
Helsinki Aging Study[66]	501	75–86	27	8.6
Redfield et al, EF by 2D visual method[2]	2036	63	—	6.0
Framingham Heart Study[3]	4257	—	44	3.0
LVSD Defined as EF <0.40				
Strong Heart Study[60]	3184	58	37	2.1
HyperGEN Study[61]	2086	55	38	3.4
Echocardiographic Heart of England Study[62]	1467	50	48	0.9
MONICA project; EF ≤0.35[67]	1467	50	48	5.9
MONICA project; EF ≤0.30[67]	1467	50	48	1.4
Redfield et al, EF by 2D visual method[2]	2036	63	—	2.0

Abbreviations: HyperGEN study, Hypertension Genetic Epidemiology Network; MONICA project, Monitoring trends and determinants of cardiovascular disease.
   [a] Based on 1698 participants.
   Adapted from Wang TJ, Levy D, Benjamin EJ, et al. The epidemiology of "asymptomatic" left ventricular systolic dysfunction: implications for screening. Ann Intern Med 2003;138:907–16; with permission.

of HF."[5] According to the guidelines, this may include previous myocardial infarction, LVSD, left ventricular hypertrophy (LVH), and valve disease. Each of these conditions may be detected by echocardiography, with generally much better sensitivity than nonimaging tools such as clinical history or electrocardiography (ECG). There is, importantly, substantial overlap as well. For instance, LVSD frequently coexists with prior myocardial infarction, valve disease, or LVH.[1,3]

Diastolic dysfunction also frequently accompanies the structural abnormalities of stage B HF. Diastolic dysfunction appears to be an important predictor of mortality in individuals after they develop symptomatic HF, regardless of etiology. For instance, Xie and colleagues[6] reported that patients with HF and restrictive filling patterns (defined as early/atrial [E/A] ratio ≥2 or E/A = 1–2, and deceleration time ≤140 milliseconds) had 1-year mortality of 19% and 2-year mortality of 51%, compared with only 5% mortality at 2 years for those with nonrestrictive diastolic filling.

Diastolic dysfunction is also common, and predicts adverse outcomes in asymptomatic individuals.[2,7] In their review of data from Olmstead County, Ammar and colleagues[8] reported that inclusion of diastolic dysfunction in the definition of stage B HF raised the percentage of individuals with this condition from 23% to 34%. Individuals with stage B HF (including diastolic dysfunction) had a 5-year survival of 96%, compared with 99% for those with no HF risk factors.

WHAT ARE THE IMPORTANT VARIABLES TO ASSESS IN THE ECHOCARDIOGRAPHIC EVALUATION?

Echocardiography is a powerful tool that provides accurate structural and functional information about the heart, without the need for ionizing radiation or intravenous contrast. A selection of the measurements that can be gathered from echocardiography to help identify those at risk of developing HF is presented in **Fig. 1**.

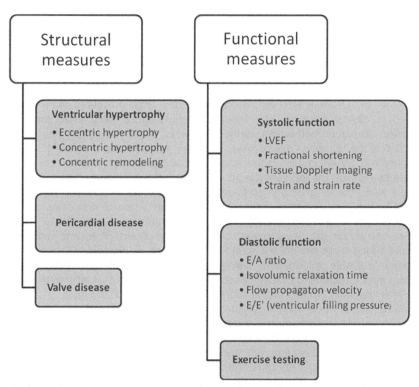

Fig. 1. Selected echocardiographic measures to use when evaluating for stage B heart failure.

LV Structure

2-Dimensional (2D) and M-mode echocardiography allow measurement of LV wall thickness in the septum (IVST) and posterior wall (PWT). Based on the thicknesses of these 2 walls and the LV internal dimension in diastole (LVIDD), left ventricular mass (LVM) can be calculated: left ventricular mass (g) = $0.8[1.04(LVIDD + IVST + PWT)^3 - (LVIDD)^3] + 0.6$.[9] LVM can be indexed according to body surface area (BSA), height, weight, and body mass index (BMI, calculated as weight in kilograms divided by height in meters squared, ie, kg/m^2). How LVM is indexed can significantly change how LVH is defined, especially in obese individuals. In a sample of obese men and women in Brazil awaiting gastric bypass surgery (average BMI 49) without any symptoms of HF, indexing LVM to body surface area yielded a prevalence of LVH of 46%, compared with as high as 82% with indexing to height alone.[10] Similarly, height indexing rather than BSA indexing resulted in a significantly higher prevalence of LVH in the community-based Framingham Heart Study.[11]

Based on wall thickness and chamber dimensions, LV geometry can also be assessed. LV geometry categories include concentric remodeling (LVM is normal and relative wall thickness [RWT, ie, the sum of the posterior and septal wall thicknesses divided by the LVIDD] is high), concentric hypertrophy (LVM and RWT are high), and eccentric hypertrophy (LVM is high but RWT is normal).[12,13] Concentric remodeling and hypertrophy are characteristic of hypertensive heart disease, whereas eccentric hypertrophy is more commonly seen in ischemic heart disease. Although it may be helpful to consider the variety of geometric abnormalities that can occur, Krumholz and colleagues[12] found that LV geometry did not add significant prognostic information once LVM and conventional risk factors were accounted for.

Systolic Function

Systolic function can be assessed quantitatively with the use of M-mode and 2D echocardiography. M-mode echocardiography allows for the measurement of linear dimensions of the left ventricle. Specifically, the LVIDD and the LV internal dimension in systole (LVIDS) can be used to calculate fractional shortening, (LVIDD − LVIDS)/LVIDD. It has been suggested that midwall fractional shortening (rather than conventional endocardial fractional shortening) provides a more physiologically accurate assessment of contractile function because the fibers responsible for short-axis shortening are located in the midwall; this is particularly important in hypertrophic, thickened walls where endocardial fractional shortening tends to overestimate systolic function.[14,15]

One-dimensional measures of LV function have obvious limitations, therefore 2D echocardiographic measures of LV function are more commonly used in clinical practice. The most commonly applied research method for determining LV function is the "Simpson rule of disks," in which an estimate of LV volume in systole and diastole is made by dividing the left ventricle into a series of disks along the long axis. In addition to these quantitative measures, qualitative assessments of LV function are often used clinically.

In populations at risk for the development of stage B HF, more subtle measures of LV dysfunction may provide valuable information. Using Doppler imaging, the LV outflow tract (LVOT) and aortic velocity-time integral (VTI) can provide information about cardiac output from the LV. Another measure is the myocardial performance index (MPI), which is derived by measuring mitral closing to opening time (a) and LV ejection time (et), and calculating the index (a − et)/et.[16] Abnormal MPI has been shown to be predictive of incident HF.[17]

Newer methods involve the use of tissue Doppler imaging (TDI). In TDI, the velocity of the myocardium itself is being measured (rather than the velocity of blood moving through the chambers as is the case in conventional Doppler). Thus, the change in the shape of the ventricle (deformation) can be measured through the cardiac cycle. Strain and its derivative, strain rate, are measures of regional deformation that have been used to assess LV systolic function. Strain and strain rate are most commonly measured in the longitudinal axis, in contrast to LVEF, which measures function along the radial axis.[18]

Diastolic Function

Diastolic function can be assessed by Doppler interrogation of transmitral inflow velocity (in early diastole [E wave] and in late diastole during atrial contraction [A wave]), tissue Doppler velocity at the mitral annulus, pulmonary venous Doppler patterns, and color M-mode flow propagation velocity. By evaluating all of these measures, an estimate of diastolic function can be obtained. In a typical grading system, diastolic dysfunction is characterized as mild (impaired relaxation), moderate (pseudonormal filling patterns), or severe (either reversible or irreversible restrictive pattern).[2,19] Impaired relaxation is characterized by reversal of transmitral E and A velocity (E/A ratio of ≤ 0.75 m/s) but normal atrial pressure

(determined by assessing mitral annular motion [e'] with TDI). A pseudonormal filling pattern refers to the apparent normalization of mitral inflow with more progressive diastolic dysfunction, with an E/A ratio greater than 0.75 m/s but less than 1.5 m/s. This pattern is typically attributed to elevation of atrial filling pressures, leading to an increase in early diastolic filling when the mitral valve first opens. In this condition, the Valsalva maneuver may unmask the reversal of E to A velocities. Finally, a restrictive (either reversible or irreversible) pattern is characterized by E/A ratios that are in excess of 1.5 m/s. Atrial pressure is very elevated when a restrictive pattern is present. Early mitral annular motion (e') typically is significantly reduced. Strain and strain rate can also be assessed in diastole, although this is done less commonly. A full description of the echocardiographic measures that determine diastolic function is presented in **Fig. 2**.

Left Atrial Size

Left atrial (LA) size can be measured either in a single dimension or by estimating 3-dimensional volume.[18] LA size is correlated with blood pressure and BMI.[20,21] LA size is associated with diastolic dysfunction, which may be attributable to LA dilation in the presence of chronically elevated filling pressures. For instance, Pritchett and colleagues[22] found that LA volume indexed to BSA increased with increasing severity of diastolic dysfunction. LA volume was predictive of mortality, but this relationship was no longer significant when adjustment for diastolic dysfunction was made.

ROLE OF ECHOCARDIOGRAPHY IN SELECTED POPULATIONS

Several populations are at higher risk of developing stage B HF, including the elderly, diabetic individuals, and those with coronary artery disease, hypertension, or obesity. Prior studies confirm a higher prevalence of echocardiographic abnormalities in these groups.

Elderly

Aurigemma and colleagues[23] studied elderly participants in the Cardiovascular Health Study who were free of HF at baseline. During a mean 5-year follow-up, 6.4% of individuals developed HF. Those who developed HF had a much higher baseline prevalence of LVH (24% in the HF group compared with 7.6% in the non-HF group), reduced systolic function (10.7% vs 5.0%), and diastolic dysfunction (average E/A ratio 0.88 vs 0.95).

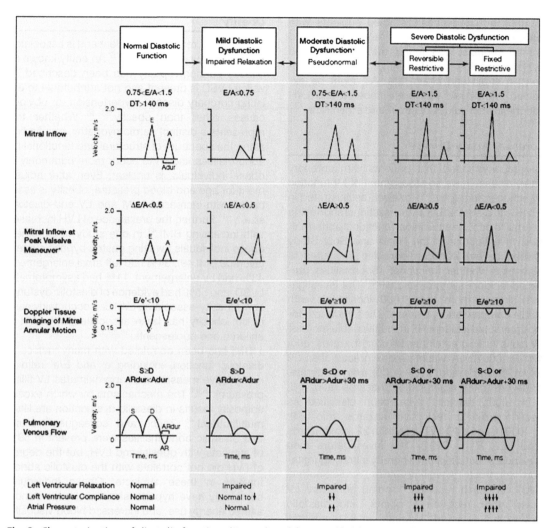

Fig. 2. Characterization of diastolic function. (*Reproduced from* Redfield MM, Jacobsen SJ, Burnett Jr JC, et al. Burden of systolic and diastolic ventricular dysfunction in the community: appreciating the scope of the heart failure epidemic. JAMA 2003;289:196; with permission.)

Diabetes

Diabetes is a major contributor to the development of LVSD and diastolic dysfunction. Certainly one reason for this is that coronary heart disease and hypertension are very common in individuals with diabetes. However, even in the absence of these conditions, diabetes is associated with an increased risk of HF, via mechanisms that are not fully understood.[24,25] The development of TDI echocardiography permits the monitoring and detection of subtle echocardiographic abnormalities that have the potential to progress to LVSD and overt HF.

Ernande and colleagues[26] assessed longitudinal and radial strain by TDI and found that both are impaired in diabetic individuals, even after

adjustment for age, sex, BMI, and other risk factors. These individuals had normal LV function by conventional echocardiographic measures of LVEF and fractional shortening. It is interesting that the diabetic individuals had reduced fractional shortening when measured at the midwall. Scholte and colleagues[27] studied 234 diabetic individuals who did not have any symptoms of HF or angina and had a normal LVEF on echocardiogram. These investigators assessed for subclinical LVSD by quantifying LV global longitudinal strain (a method that calculates longitudinal strain values from all 17 segments of the left ventricle and averages them). Individuals with impaired global longitudinal strain were more likely to have coronary atherosclerosis (identified by coronary artery calcium scoring).

Fang and colleagues[28] studied subjects with diabetes, diabetes and LVH, LVH alone, and normal controls, and found that diabetes and LVH were each associated with significant reductions in strain and strain rate. As might be expected, individuals with both diabetes and LVH had the lowest values of strain and strain rate.

Coronary Artery Disease

It is recommended that patients with coronary artery disease have an assessment of LV function by echocardiography.[29] However, as illustrated in those with diabetes, LVEF and fractional shortening may fail to capture subclinical functional abnormalities. Investigators in the Heart and Soul Study studied several echocardiographic measures to determine whether functional abnormalities predicted incident symptomatic HF.[30] The investigators studied more than 1000 individuals with stable coronary artery disease. The following findings predicted incident HF in multivariable models: LV mass index greater than 90 g/m^2 (hazards ratio, 4.1; P<.0001), LA volume index greater than 29 mL/m^2 (hazards ratio, 1.6; P = .06), mild, moderate, or severe mitral regurgitation (hazards ratio, 1.8; P = .009), diastolic dysfunction classified as pseudonormal or restrictive (hazards ratio, 2.9; $P \leq$.0001), and LVOT VTI less than 22 mm (hazards ratio, 2.2; P = .0004). The investigators then created a scoring system whereby mitral regurgitation, abnormal LA volume index, and abnormal LVOT VTI each received 1 point, abnormal LV mass index received 3 points, and diastolic dysfunction received 2 points. In 831 subjects with no history of HF, 39% of those with a score of 7 to 8 (the highest score, assigned to 4% of individuals overall) developed HF during follow-up. By contrast, only 3% of those with scores totaling 0 to 2 experienced an incident HF event. Subjects with the highest scores were at statistically significantly increased risk of HF even after adjusting for age, size of prior MI, LVEF, and a host of other clinical risk factors including N-terminal pro–B-type natriuretic peptide (NT-proBNP).

In individuals with established coronary artery disease, diastolic dysfunction is common and carries a significant risk of incident HF. Ren and colleagues[31] studied a population of 693 patients with stable coronary artery disease but no evidence of reduced LVEF or symptoms of HF. Overall, 24% of the sample had mild diastolic dysfunction by echocardiography, and 10% had moderate to severe diastolic dysfunction. Moderate to severe diastolic dysfunction was associated with a hazards ratio of 6.3 (95% confidence interval, 2.4–16.1) for HF hospitalization.

Obesity

Obesity is increasingly prevalent and is associated with an increased risk of HF.[32] An entity known as obesity cardiomyopathy has been described, in which LVSD is present and not attributable to existing coronary disease, hypertension, or obvious causes other than obesity.[33–36] Whether this represents a distinct cardiomyopathy, or a finding along the spectrum of structural and functional LV abnormalities known to occur more commonly in obese individuals, is unclear. Even after adjustment for age and blood pressure, obesity is associated with increased LVM and LV end-diastolic size.[37–41] Further, the prevalence of LVH increases with increasing BMI.[41] In one study of extremely obese individuals awaiting gastric bypass surgery (average BMI 49), 54% had left atrial enlargement, 43% had LV enlargement, 11% had asymptomatic LVSD, and 55% had evidence of diastolic dysfunction. Obesity-associated LVH can occur fairly early in life; obesity has been associated with LVH in children and adolescents.[38,39,42]

BMI has been correlated with many indices of diastolic function, including e' and E/e' ratio (a noninvasive measure that approximates LV filling pressure).[43,44] The mechanisms by which excess adiposity results in diastolic dysfunction are likely multifactorial.[45] Zarich and colleagues[45] found that diastolic abnormalities were present in 50% of subjects with obesity and LVH, but the degree of LVH did not correlate with the diastolic abnormalities in these subjects. Obese individuals commonly have hypertension, insulin resistance, altered energy use, and increased blood viscosity, all of which may contribute to LV diastolic dysfunction.[46,47]

Whatever mechanisms are involved in obesity-association LVH and LV dysfunction, weight loss can reverse many of the changes. In a study of 423 obese subjects who underwent gastric bypass surgery, LVM decreased by about 14% at 2 years after surgery, and midwall fractional shortening increased, supporting the hypothesis that weight loss improves LV structure and function.[48]

Hypertension

Hypertension is a major risk factor for HF. It is also well known to be associated with LVH and abnormalities of both diastolic and systolic dysfunction.[49] In a study of 2384 subjects with untreated hypertension, asymptomatic LVSD was present in 3.6%. The annual incidence of HF per 100 persons in the LVSD group was 1.48, compared with only 0.12 in the normal LV systolic function group (P<.0001). In a multivariable-adjusted model, the hazards ratio for development of HF was 9.99 ($P = .0001$).[50]

Subtle abnormalities in systolic function can be detected in hypertensive individuals using TDI technology. In a study of 92 asymptomatic hypertensive subjects with normal LVEF, 10% were found to have impaired systolic function as measured by TDI. The investigators also found that there was a strong correlation ($r = 0.67$, $P<.0001$) between systolic and diastolic annular velocities, suggesting that diastolic and systolic function tracked together.[51] That impaired systolic function may be present in diastolic HF is important to consider when defining a therapeutic strategy for these individuals.

COST EFFECTIVENESS AND HANDHELD ECHOCARDIOGRAPHY

Although echocardiography is the most commonly used modality for assessing systolic and diastolic function, its use as a screening tool in the general population may be limited by cost. Some have suggested that echocardiography be used as a second step in screening,[52] after less expensive clinical assessment and biochemical analyses. The family of natriuretic peptides (BNP, NT-proBNP) are the most commonly used biomarkers to monitor and diagnose chronic HF, and thus a possible choice as a screening biomarker.

Several groups have assessed different combination strategies for identifying people with asymptomatic LVSD. Heidenreich and colleagues[53] performed a cost-effectiveness analysis comparing a "no screening" strategy with "BNP then echo," "BNP alone," and "Echo alone" strategies. For men, the "BNP then echo strategy" cost $22,300 per quality-adjusted life year (QALY), compared with $123,500 for echocardiography alone. Because the prevalence of asymptomatic LVSD is much lower in women, most screening strategies for asymptomatic LVSD do not seem cost effective in this group. For women, the "BNP then echo" strategy had an incremental cost effectiveness of $77,700. The investigators performed a sensitivity analysis considering different prevalence rates of asymptomatic LVSD. Not unexpectedly, for both men and women cost effectiveness dropped significantly as prevalence decreased.[53] Thus, focusing screening programs on individuals who are at highest risk for developing LVSD (those with diabetes, hypertension, prior coronary disease, or obesity) may significantly improve the attractiveness of echocardiographic screening strategies.

Less costly methods of imaging may also improve cost effectiveness. Handheld ultrasound units are far less expensive than standard echocardiography machines, and appear to generate comparable measures of LV structure and function.[54–58] To compare the 2 technologies, Prinz and Voigt[59] compared results from handheld echocardiography (HHE) with high-end standard echocardiography in 349 individuals. Regional wall motion ($\kappa = 0.73$, $P<.01$), LV measurements ($r = 0.99$, $P<.01$), and valvular regurgitation ($\kappa = 0.9$, $P<.01$) showed high degrees of concordance between HHE and standard echocardiography. A high degree of correlation between traditional echocardiography and HHE was also found in another study of 531 individuals drawn from a community-based HF screening program. The correlation coefficient for LVEF was 0.9, and HHE had a sensitivity of 96% and a specificity of 98% for the detection of asymptomatic LVSD (when using standard echocardiography as the gold standard). These results were similar between high-risk groups and the general population.[57]

These investigators also performed a cost-effectiveness analysis comparing 7 different screening strategies with HHE or traditional echocardiography for the detection of asymptomatic LVSD, and compared the cost of each strategy in low-risk, intermediate-risk, and high-risk populations. The least effective strategy was screening low-risk people with traditional echocardiography alone (cost per case of asymptomatic LVSD found, $90,278) whereas the most cost-effective strategy was screening high-risk individuals (those with ischemic heart disease, diabetes, hypertension, peripheral vascular disease, cerebrovascular disease, or heavy alcohol use) using a strategy that involved initial screening with an ECG. Under this approach, an abnormal ECG was followed up with HHE first, then traditional echocardiography. This strategy cost $915 per case of asymptomatic LVSD identified. By comparison, screening with traditional echocardiography alone in the high-risk population cost $2476.[56]

These studies suggest that screening for asymptomatic LVSD with echocardiography may be cost effective if 2 criteria are met: (1) screening is restricted to high-risk populations, and (2) the screening strategy involves a phased approach whereby the most expensive technology is used only after less expensive tests have demonstrated an abnormality.

SUMMARY

As greater emphasis is placed on prevention of symptomatic HF, accurate and cost-effective strategies to identify stage B HF become critical. Echocardiography is a well-established and effective tool for identifying most abnormalities associated with stage B HF. Cost-effectiveness analyses suggest that targeting echocardiography to selected individuals, after an initial clinical assessment, could be a promising approach to screening. Expanded use of newer technologies, including TDI and HHE, could improve the efficiency of these strategies even further.

REFERENCES

1. Wang TJ, Levy D, Benjamin EJ, et al. The epidemiology of "asymptomatic" left ventricular systolic dysfunction: implications for screening. Ann Intern Med 2003;138:907–16.
2. Redfield MM, Jacobsen SJ, Burnett JC Jr, et al. Burden of systolic and diastolic ventricular dysfunction in the community: appreciating the scope of the heart failure epidemic. JAMA 2003;289:194–202.
3. Wang TJ, Evans JC, Benjamin EJ, et al. Natural history of asymptomatic left ventricular systolic dysfunction in the community. Circulation 2003;108:977–82.
4. Effect of enalapril on survival in patients with reduced left ventricular ejection fractions and congestive heart failure. The SOLVD Investigators. N Engl J Med 1991;325:293–302.
5. Hunt SA, Baker DW, Chin MH, et al. ACC/AHA Guidelines for the Evaluation and Management of Chronic Heart Failure in the Adult: Executive Summary A Report of the American College of Cardiology/American Heart Association Task Force on Practice Guidelines (Committee to Revise the 1995 Guidelines for the Evaluation and Management of Heart Failure): Developed in Collaboration With the International Society for Heart and Lung Transplantation; Endorsed by the Heart Failure Society of America. Circulation 2001;104:2996–3007.
6. Xie GY, Berk MR, Smith MD, et al. Prognostic value of Doppler transmitral flow patterns in patients with congestive heart failure. J Am Coll Cardiol 1994; 24:132–9.
7. Bella JN, Palmieri V, Roman MJ, et al. Mitral ratio of peak early to late diastolic filling velocity as a predictor of mortality in middle-aged and elderly adults: the Strong Heart Study. Circulation 2002;105:1928–33.
8. Ammar KA, Jacobsen SJ, Mahoney DW, et al. Prevalence and prognostic significance of heart failure stages: application of the American College of Cardiology/American Heart Association heart failure staging criteria in the community. Circulation 2007; 115:1563–70.
9. Devereux RB, Alonso DR, Lutas EM, et al. Echocardiographic assessment of left ventricular hypertrophy: comparison to necropsy findings. Am J Cardiol 1986;57:450–8.
10. Rocha IE, Victor EG, Braga MC, et al. Echocardiography evaluation for asymptomatic patients with severe obesity. Arq Bras Cardiol 2007;88:52–8.
11. Levy D, Savage DD, Garrison RJ, et al. Echocardiographic criteria for left ventricular hypertrophy: the Framingham Heart Study. Am J Cardiol 1987;59: 956–60.
12. Krumholz HM, Larson M, Levy D. Prognosis of left ventricular geometric patterns in the Framingham Heart Study. J Am Coll Cardiol 1995;25:879–84.
13. Velagaleti RS, Gona P, Levy D, et al. Relations of biomarkers representing distinct biological pathways to left ventricular geometry. Circulation 2008; 118:2252–8, 5p following 2258.
14. de Simone G, Devereux RB, Roman MJ, et al. Assessment of left ventricular function by the midwall fractional shortening/end-systolic stress relation in human hypertension. J Am Coll Cardiol 1994;23: 1444–51.
15. Ballo P, Mondillo S, Motto A, et al. Left ventricular midwall mechanics in subjects with aortic stenosis and normal systolic chamber function. J Heart Valve Dis 2006;15:639–50.
16. Tei C, Ling LH, Hodge DO, et al. New index of combined systolic and diastolic myocardial performance: a simple and reproducible measure of cardiac function—a study in normals and dilated cardiomyopathy. J Cardiol 1995;26:357–66.
17. Arnlov J, Ingelsson E, Riserus U, et al. Myocardial performance index, a Doppler-derived index of global left ventricular function, predicts congestive heart failure in elderly men. Eur Heart J 2004;25: 2220–5.
18. Armstrong WR, Ryan T. Feigenbaum's echocardiography. 7th edition. Philadelphia: Lippincott Williams and Wilkins; 2010.
19. Nishimura RA, Tajik AJ. Evaluation of diastolic filling of left ventricle in health and disease: Doppler echocardiography is the clinician's Rosetta Stone. J Am Coll Cardiol 1997;30:8–18.
20. McManus DD, Xanthakis V, Sullivan LM, et al. Longitudinal tracking of left atrial diameter over the adult life course: clinical correlates in the community. Circulation 2010;121:667–74.
21. Stritzke J, Markus MR, Duderstadt S, et al. The aging process of the heart: obesity is the main risk factor for left atrial enlargement during aging the MONICA/KORA (monitoring of trends and determinations in cardiovascular disease/cooperative research in the region of Augsburg) study. J Am Coll Cardiol 2009; 54:1982–9.
22. Pritchett AM, Mahoney DW, Jacobsen SJ, et al. Diastolic dysfunction and left atrial volume: a population-based study. J Am Coll Cardiol 2005;45: 87–92.
23. Aurigemma GP, Gottdiener JS, Shemanski L, et al. Predictive value of systolic and diastolic function for incident congestive heart failure in the elderly: the cardiovascular health study. J Am Coll Cardiol 2001;37:1042–8.

24. Ahmed SS, Jaferi GA, Narang RM, et al. Preclinical abnormality of left ventricular function in diabetes mellitus. Am Heart J 1975;89:153–8.

25. Boudina S, Abel ED. Diabetic cardiomyopathy revisited. Circulation 2007;115:3213–23.

26. Ernande L, Rietzschel ER, Bergerot C, et al. Impaired myocardial radial function in asymptomatic patients with type 2 diabetes mellitus: a speckle-tracking imaging study. J Am Soc Echocardiogr 2010;23:1266–72.

27. Scholte AJ, Nucifora G, Delgado V, et al. Subclinical left ventricular dysfunction and coronary atherosclerosis in asymptomatic patients with type 2 diabetes. Eur J Echocardiogr 2011;12(2):148–55.

28. Fang ZY, Yuda S, Anderson V, et al. Echocardiographic detection of early diabetic myocardial disease. J Am Coll Cardiol 2003;41:611–7.

29. Cheitlin MD, Alpert JS, Armstrong WF, et al. ACC/AHA Guidelines for the Clinical Application of Echocardiography. A report of the American College of Cardiology/American Heart Association Task Force on Practice Guidelines (Committee on Clinical Application of Echocardiography). Developed in collaboration with the American Society of Echocardiography. Circulation 1997;95:1686–744.

30. Stevens SM, Farzaneh-Far R, Na B, et al. Development of an echocardiographic risk-stratification index to predict heart failure in patients with stable coronary artery disease: the Heart and Soul study. JACC Cardiovasc Imaging 2009;2:11–20.

31. Ren X, Ristow B, Na B, et al. Prevalence and prognosis of asymptomatic left ventricular diastolic dysfunction in ambulatory patients with coronary heart disease. Am J Cardiol 2007;99:1643–7.

32. Clark K. Obesity and the risk of heart failure. J Insur Med 2003;35:59–60.

33. Wang Y, Hu G. Individual and joint associations of obesity and physical activity on the risk of heart failure. Congest Heart Fail 2010;16:292–9.

34. Kenchaiah S, Gaziano JM, Vasan RS. Impact of obesity on the risk of heart failure and survival after the onset of heart failure. Med Clin North Am 2004; 88:1273–94.

35. Horwich TB, Fonarow GC. Glucose, obesity, metabolic syndrome, and diabetes relevance to incidence of heart failure. J Am Coll Cardiol 2010;55: 283–93.

36. Baena-Diez JM, Byram AO, Grau M, et al. Obesity is an independent risk factor for heart failure: Zona Franca Cohort study. Clin Cardiol 2010;33: 760–4.

37. Chadha DS, Gupta N, Goel K, et al. Impact of obesity on the left ventricular functions and morphology of healthy Asian Indians. Metab Syndr Relat Disord 2009;7:151–8.

38. Movahed MR, Martinez A, Greaves J, et al. Left ventricular hypertrophy is associated with obesity, male gender, and symptoms in healthy adolescents. Obesity (Silver Spring) 2009;17:606–10.

39. Movahed MR, Bates S, Strootman D, et al. Obesity in adolescence is associated with left ventricular hypertrophy and hypertension. Echocardiography 2011;28:150–3.

40. Guerra F, Mancinelli L, Angelini L, et al. The association of left ventricular hypertrophy with metabolic syndrome is dependent on body mass index in hypertensive overweight or obese patients. PLoS One 2011;6:e16630.

41. Lauer MS, Anderson KM, Kannel WB, et al. The impact of obesity on left ventricular mass and geometry. The Framingham Heart Study. JAMA 1991;266: 231–6.

42. Chinali M, de Simone G, Roman MJ, et al. Impact of obesity on cardiac geometry and function in a population of adolescents: the Strong Heart Study. J Am Coll Cardiol 2006;47:2267–73.

43. Russo C, Jin Z, Homma S, et al. Effect of obesity and overweight on left ventricular diastolic function a community-based study in an elderly cohort. J Am Coll Cardiol 2011;57:1368–74.

44. Hillis GS, Moller JE, Pellikka PA, et al. Noninvasive estimation of left ventricular filling pressure by E/e' is a powerful predictor of survival after acute myocardial infarction. J Am Coll Cardiol 2004;43: 360–7.

45. Zarich SW, Kowalchuk GJ, McGuire MP, et al. Left ventricular filling abnormalities in asymptomatic morbid obesity. Am J Cardiol 1991;68:377–81.

46. von Haehling S, Doehner W, Anker SD. Obesity and the heart a weighty issue. J Am Coll Cardiol 2006;47: 2274–6.

47. Marin-Garcia J, Goldenthal MJ. Fatty acid metabolism in cardiac failure: biochemical, genetic and cellular analysis. Cardiovasc Res 2002;54:516–27.

48. Owan T, Avelar E, Morley K, et al. Favorable changes in cardiac geometry and function following gastric bypass surgery: 2-year follow-up in the Utah obesity study. J Am Coll Cardiol 2011;57:732–9.

49. Volpe M, McKelvie R, Drexler H. Hypertension as an underlying factor in heart failure with preserved ejection fraction. J Clin Hypertens (Greenwich) 2010;12: 277–83.

50. Verdecchia P, Angeli F, Gattobigio R, et al. Asymptomatic left ventricular systolic dysfunction in essential hypertension: prevalence, determinants, and prognostic value. Hypertension 2005;45:412–8.

51. Nishikage T, Nakai H, Lang RM, et al. Subclinical left ventricular longitudinal systolic dysfunction in hypertension with no evidence of heart failure. Circ J 2008; 72:189–94.

52. Colonna P, Pinto FJ, Sorino M, et al. The emerging role of echocardiography in the screening of patients at risk of heart failure. Am J Cardiol 2005; 96:42L–51L.

53. Heidenreich PA, Gubens MA, Fonarow GC, et al. Cost-effectiveness of screening with B-type natriuretic peptide to identify patients with reduced left ventricular ejection fraction. J Am Coll Cardiol 2004;43:1019–26.

54. Hebert K, Horswell R, Heidenreich P, et al. Handheld ultrasound, B-natriuretic peptide for screening stage B heart failure. South Med J 2010;103:616–22.

55. Atherton JJ. Screening for left ventricular systolic dysfunction: is imaging a solution? JACC Cardiovasc Imaging 2010;3:121–8.

56. Galasko GI, Barnes SC, Collinson P, et al. What is the most cost-effective strategy to screen for left ventricular systolic dysfunction: natriuretic peptides, the electrocardiogram, hand-held echocardiography, traditional echocardiography, or their combination? Eur Heart J 2006;27:193–200.

57. Galasko GI, Lahiri A, Senior R. Portable echocardiography: an innovative tool in screening for cardiac abnormalities in the community. Eur J Echocardiogr 2003;4:119–27.

58. Vourvouri EC, Schinkel AF, Roelandt JR, et al. Screening for left ventricular dysfunction using a hand-carried cardiac ultrasound device. Eur J Heart Fail 2003;5:767–74.

59. Prinz C, Voigt JU. Diagnostic accuracy of a handheld ultrasound scanner in routine patients referred for echocardiography. J Am Soc Echocardiogr 2011;24:111–6.

60. Devereux RB, Roman MJ, Paranicas M, et al. A population-based assessment of left ventricular systolic dysfunction in middle-aged and older adults: the Strong Heart Study. Am Heart J 2001; 141:439–46.

61. Devereux RB, Bella JN, Palmieri V, et al. Left ventricular systolic dysfunction in a biracial sample of hypertensive adults: The Hypertension Genetic Epidemiology Network (HyperGEN) Study. Hypertension 2001;38:417–23.

62. Davies M, Hobbs F, Davis R, et al. Prevalence of left-ventricular systolic dysfunction and heart failure in the Echocardiographic Heart of England Screening study: a population based study. Lancet 2001;358: 439–44.

63. Schunkert H, Broeckel U, Hense HW, et al. Left-ventricular dysfunction. Lancet 1998;351:372.

64. Hedberg P, Lonnberg I, Jonason T, et al. Left ventricular systolic dysfunction in 75-year-old men and women; a population-based study. Eur Heart J 2001;22:676–83.

65. Mosterd A, Hoes AW, de Bruyne MC, et al. Prevalence of heart failure and left ventricular dysfunction in the general population; The Rotterdam Study. Eur Heart J 1999;20:447–55.

66. Kupari M, Lindroos M, Iivanainen AM, et al. Congestive heart failure in old age: prevalence, mechanisms and 4-year prognosis in the Helsinki Ageing Study. J Intern Med 1997;241:387–94.

67. McDonagh TA, Morrison CE, Lawrence A, et al. Symptomatic and asymptomatic left-ventricular systolic dysfunction in an urban population. Lancet 1997;350:829–33.

Cardiac Magnetic Resonance Imaging for Stage B Heart Failure

Sara L. Partington, MD[a,b], Susan Cheng, MD[c],
João A.C. Lima, MD[d,e],*

KEYWORDS

- Cardiac MRI • Heart failure • Stage B heart failure

Cardiac imaging plays an essential role in the assessment of patients with heart failure (HF) at all stages of disease. However, cardiac imaging may have the most to offer individuals with stage B disease, defined as the presence of asymptomatic cardiac structure or functional abnormalities, because these patients stand to substantially benefit from early interventions before the onset of overt HF. As such, cardiac magnetic resonance (CMR) imaging can serve as a particularly important imaging modality for providing both diagnostic and prognostic information in the setting of stage B disease. CMR is already considered the reference standard for conventional measurements of left and right ventricular structure and systolic function.[1] In addition, CMR allows for detailed myocardial tissue characterization, which can aid clinicians in identifying the cause of a given cardiomyopathy. Furthermore, CMR techniques can be used to quantify variations in regional and global myocardial performance, even in the presence of a normal ejection fraction (EF). In turn, both conventional and novel CMR measures of cardiac structure and function can be used to estimate prognosis and could also serve as potential targets of therapy.

CARDIAC MAGNETIC RESONANCE IMAGING FOR HEART FAILURE: TECHNICAL CONSIDERATIONS

Multiple imaging modalities are available for assessing cardiac structure and function in the setting of HF. The unique and complementary role of CMR can be appreciated in the context of several technical considerations.

Advantages

It remains widely recognized that CMR provides the most precise and reproducible noninvasive assessment of cardiac systolic function. Compared with echocardiography, CMR offers the advantage of excellent visualization of the endocardial border in addition to high spatial resolution

Disclosures: The authors have no relevant conflicts.
a Non-Invasive Cardiovascular Imaging Program, Department of Medicine, Brigham and Women's Hospital, 75 Francis Street, Boston, MA 02115, USA
b Non-Invasive Cardiovascular Imaging Program, Department of Radiology, Brigham and Women's Hospital, 75 Francis Street, Boston, MA 02115, USA
c Division of Cardiovascular Medicine, Department of Medicine, Brigham and Women's Hospital, 75 Francis Street, Boston, MA 02115, USA
d Department of Medicine, Johns Hopkins School of Medicine and Johns Hopkins Hospital, Baltimore, MD, USA
e Department of Radiology, Johns Hopkins School of Medicine and Johns Hopkins Hospital, Baltimore, MD, USA
* Corresponding author. Division of Cardiology, Johns Hopkins Hospital, Blalock 524D Cardiology Division, 600 North Wolfe Street, Blalock 524, Baltimore, MD 21287.
E-mail address: jlima@jhmi.edu

Heart Failure Clin 8 (2012) 179–190
doi:10.1016/j.hfc.2011.11.009
1551-7136/12/$ – see front matter © 2012 Published by Elsevier Inc.

(up to 1.5 mm × 1.5 mm in plane resolution), without the limitation of poor echo windows. In addition, CMR-based assessments of left ventricular (LV) architecture do not require geometric assumptions. These features lead to very high intrareader and inter-reader reproducibility when assessing LV volumes and LVEF, with coefficients of variation less than 5%.[2] Such low variability makes CMR particularly valuable for serial follow-up evaluations of the same patient. The combination of high spatial resolution and low variability can be especially important in clinical settings whereby a precise cutoff value for a given therapy is required, such as for evaluating LVEF in patients being considered for implantable cardiac defibrillator (ICD) therapy.

In addition to providing precise and highly reproducible assessments of EF, CMR offers several additional technical advantages: CMR is currently the only noninvasive imaging modality that can be used for myocardial tissue characterization; standard assessment of cardiac structure and function, in addition to tissue characterization, can be performed within a single study that can be completed in less than 1 hour; and, compared with radiograph-based imaging modalities, CMR does not use ionizing radiation, which is favorable in younger patients or patients in need of repeat imaging.

Limitations

Notwithstanding the advantages of CMR, several limitations merit consideration. In patients with severe kidney failure, gadolinium-containing contrast agents pose the risk of nephrogenic systemic fibrosis (NSF). NSF results in bilateral, fibrotic, indurated papules; plaques; and subcutaneous nodules commonly involving the extremities. The fibrosis may be sufficiently severe to cause flexion contractures, joint immobility, pain, paresthesias, and severe puritis. Systemic involvement resulting in muscle induration; joint contracture; or fibrosis of the lung, myocardium, pericardium, or pleura has also been reported.[3] Although the symptoms are disabling and not treatable, NSF is rare and occurs exclusively in patients with kidney failure, with most cases involving patients with advanced kidney disease (dialysis or a glomerular filtration rate <30 mL/min),[4] acute kidney injury,[5] or those hospitalized for a proinflammatory event.[5]

Preventing NSF involves avoiding gadolinium-containing contrast in higher-risk patients. In cases whereby the benefits of administering gadolinium outweigh the risks and adequate diagnostic information cannot be obtained with a noncontrast study, decreasing the gadolinium dose to the lowest dose deemed necessary (ie, single dose [0.1 mmol/Kg] rather than double dose [0.2 mmol/Kg]) may reduce the risk.[6] Although NSF is presumed to occur with any gadolinium-containing contrast agent, most reported cases of NSF have occurred using gadodiamide,[5,6] a contrast agent that contains a chelating agent that less tightly binds gadolinium. Thus, the overall risk may be decreased by using a gadolinium formulation with a tighter-binding chelating agent (eg, gadoteridol). In renal patients without alternative imaging options, the overall risk for NSF may be further reduced by performing dialysis within 12 to 24 hours after gadolinium exposure.

The presence of a pacemaker or ICD currently remains a contraindication to CMR. Growing evidence suggests that patients with pacemakers manufactured in recent years can undergo CMR safely when a modified magnetic resonance imaging (MRI) pulse sequence protocol is used under close supervision in an experienced center. Recently, MRI-compatible pacemakers have been manufactured and clinical trials of these devices are underway to assess safety.

Even in the absence of internal cardiac devices, CMR remains challenging in patients with irregular heart rhythms or with difficultly holding their breath. Modified sequences that are less sensitive to cardiac gating and respiratory motion can compensate for some of these challenges. However, some of these modified sequences are longer in duration and can result in reduced image quality.

ASSESSMENT OF LEFT VENTRICULAR FUNCTION

In the presence of abnormal cardiac structure, it is important to obtain an accurate assessment of associated cardiac function. Although common manifestations of LV remodeling are known to increase an individual's overall risk for cardiovascular events, the presence of asymptomatic LV dysfunction, even when mild, is particularly associated with the development of clinical HF as well as all-cause death.[7]

The standard metric of global systolic function remains the LVEF. CMR provides the reference standard assessment of LVEF given its excellent temporal resolution, spatial resolution, and tissue contrast abilities differentiating the endocardial border from the blood pool.[8] Cine movie images to assess LV systolic function are most often performed with steady state free precession (SSFP) imaging by displaying the same myocardial slice at different points within the cardiac cycle. The systolic and diastolic cavities can be traced in multiple contiguous short-axis images of the LV cavity (typically at 1-cm intervals) starting at the mitral valve level and moving toward the LV apex. An accurate assessment of LVEF can be made using Simpson's rule (**Fig. 1**). Because contiguous slices of the heart are obtained, no geometric assumptions regarding of the shape of the heart are required, such as when performing 3-dimensional models to calculate volumes by echocardiography, which is particularly valuable in patients with HF with ischemic cardiomyopathy and focal wall motion abnormalities. A lack of geometric assumptions is also important in the setting of dilated cardiomyopathy because as the heart dilates, the LV becomes more spherical and the relationship between length and diameter is altered.[9]

Another possible role for CMR in patients with stage B HF is the assessment of diastolic function. The importance of evaluating diastolic function is underscored by the fact that approximately half of patients presenting with clinical HF have preserved EF.[10] Although echocardiography remains the standard modality of assessing diastolic function, novel CMR techniques can also provide useful information about myocardial performance in diastole. As with echocardiography, mitral valve early diastolic flow (*E*) and atrial contraction flow (*A*) can be measured using CMR phase contrast imaging, which assesses the velocity and volume of blood flow throughout the cardiac cycle. That said, CMR phase contrast does tend to overestimate *A* velocity compared with Doppler echocardiography,[11] and the calculation of the *E/A* ratio is intrinsically limited because the *E* filling velocity depends on left atrial pressure leading to pseudonormalization of the *E/A* ratio in patients with elevated left atrial pressure and impaired diastolic filling. However, novel CMR sequences have been developed to assess

the motion of moving structures through tissue phase contrast, similar to tissue Doppler in echocardiography, allowing for the measurement of early mitral septal tissue velocity (*Ea*) and the calculation of the *E/Ea* ratio. Both echocardiographic and CMR methods for estimating the *E/Ea* ratio have good correlation with pulmonary capillary wedge measurements, although the correlation for Doppler echocardiography is slightly better (r = 0.85 compared with 0.80).[11] Nonetheless, CMR is a viable option for the evaluation of diastolic function in patients with poor echo windows.

DETERMINING CAUSE

For the purposes of defining cause, a unique property of CMR is its ability to provide detailed myocardial tissue characterization in a way that can aid the clinician in determining the causes or pathogenesis of a given cardiomyopathy. To this end, CMR can be used to assess the presence versus absence of several key characteristics that may be involved in a particular disease process, including inflammation, fibrosis, scar, ischemia, and viability. An overall assessment of these characteristics can be used to determine the likelihood that asymptomatic cardiac abnormalities are caused by ischemic versus nonischemic pathologic conditions, which has bearing on prognosis and therapy.

Several CMR techniques can be used to aid in determining the cause of a given cardiomyopathy. By using specialized CMR pulse sequences, myocardium can be clearly differentiated from fat and fluid. In turn, regions of myocardial inflammation can be identified using T2-weighted imaging, given the higher associated fluid content in these specific areas of myocardial tissue. Similarly, regions of edema can be seen in active myocarditis as well as in some infiltrative

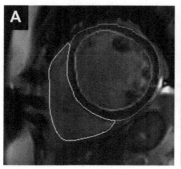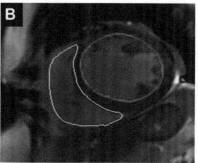

Fig. 1. SSFP image of the short axis of the LV at papillary muscle level demonstrating the LV diastolic volume (*A*) and LV systolic volume (*B*) to quantify the LVEF by Simpson's rule.

cardiomyopathies that can involve active inflammation, such as sarcoidosis. Gadolinium–diethylenetriamine pentaacetic acid can be administered to patients during the study that distributes to areas of myocardial blood flow, and perfusion can be assessed. Gadolinium is extracellular and resides in the interstitial space of territories that receive myocardial blood flow. Territories with scar have significant replacement fibrosis and more interstitial space and, as a result, they concentrate gadolinium.

Late gadolinium enhancement (LGE) is probably the most widely used and investigated CMR technique for determining cause and prognosis in the setting of cardiomyopathy. Initially developed as an extension of experimental studies using iodinated contrast imaged by computed tomography,[12] it suffered in the beginning from the poor temporal resolution of cardiac MRI based on early spin echo techniques.[13] Only after the development of gradient echo MRI pulse sequences, infarct necrosis could be distinguished from superimposed regions of microvascular obstruction.[14,15] Later pulse sequence development with the introduction of inversion recovery techniques led

to methodology currently used clinically.[16] At present, LGE sequences obtained approximately 10 minutes after gadolinium injection allow time for gadolinium to both concentrate in regions of increased interstitial space or penetrate cells with disrupted membranes and to clear from the blood pool. The result is a distinct contrast between the amount of gadolinium concentrated in the heart versus amount of gadolinium in the blood. Because gadolinium has magnetic properties that are unique from the magnetic properties of blood or myocardium, the increased gadolinium content in areas of scar become enhanced when specific strongly T1-weighted pulse sequences are performed. Normal myocardium is set to appear black (Fig. 2A) with regions of gadolinium accumulation appearing white. Enhanced (white) regions indicate areas of gadolinium accumulation and suggest the presence of inflammation, fibrosis, or scar. Alternatively, such regions could represent an expansion of the myocardial interstitium that develops as a result of an infiltrative process. The ease with which LGE can be assessed has improved since the development of rapid sequences for detecting LGE. Thus, if

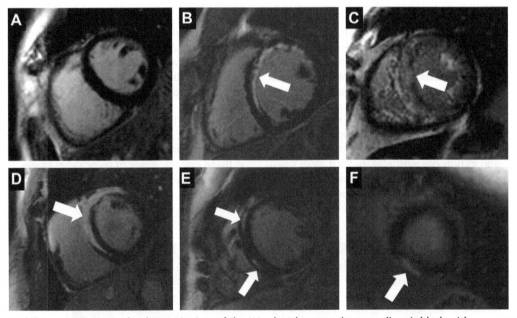

Fig. 2. (A) An LGE image in the short-axis view of the LV, whereby normal myocardium is black with no areas of hyperenhancement (white) to suggest scar, fibrosis, or expansion of the myocardial interstitium as in an infiltrative cardiomyopathy. (B) An ischemic cardiomyopathy with subendocardial LGE in the anterior, anteroseptal, and inferoseptal walls (arrow) consistent with a myocardial infarction of the left anterior descending coronary artery. (C) The short axis demonstrating cardiac amyloid with increased LV mass and global subendocardial LGE (arrow). Note that the blood pool is dark because of the rapid removal of gadolinium from blood into amyloid infiltrated organs. (D) Bright epicardial enhancement in the anterior, septal, and right ventricular walls, indicating active cardiac sarcoid granulomatous infiltration (arrow). (E) A dilated nonischemic cardiomyopathy with typical midwall LGE (arrows). (F) Subepicardial hyperenhancement (arrow) consistent with active myocarditis.

required, images can be obtained without the need for patients to hold their breath or even have a regular cardiac rhythm.[17]

Patterns of Disease

The specific pattern of tissue characteristics is often quite informative with respect to identifying either an ischemic or nonischemic cause underlying a given cardiomyopathy. In ischemic cardiomyopathy, the presence of coronary artery disease (CAD) is characterized by the presence of subendocardial to transmural LGE in anatomic regions corresponding to territories of coronary artery perfusion distribution (see **Fig. 2**B). The typical subendocardial location of the scar derives from the fact that the coronary arteries typically course along the epicardium and, in the setting of hemodynamically significant stenoses, the endocardium is the most vulnerable to deprivation of blood flow at the time of a myocardial infarction (MI).[18]

The combination of LGE pattern and additional CMR tissue characteristics can also be informative regarding nonischemic causes. For example, cardiac amyloidosis frequently demonstrates diffuse global subendocardial LGE (see **Fig. 2**C) and occasionally atrial enhancement. In many patients with heavy systemic amyloid burden, the speed of contrast washout from the blood pool increases substantially, compared with typical patients, because of the increased myocardial uptake of gadolinium into the increased interstitial space resulting from the amyloid infiltration into the myocardium. Because of this phenomenon, LGE images should be acquired earlier, starting 5 minutes after gadolinium administration, in patients with a suspicion of cardiac amyloid.[19] Patients with Chagas heart disease, which is frequently in the differential diagnosis of patients with suspected sarcoidosis, develop myocardial fibrosis that can be quantified by MRI. Asymptomatic patients with Chagas disease, who generally have conduction abnormalities such as right bundle branch block (RBBB) with left anterior fasicular block (LAFB), have less fibrosis than patients with symptomatic disease.[20]

In contrast to the typically diffuse LGE pattern of amyloid, cardiac sarcoidosis usually demonstrates patchy LGE in the myocardium of either the LV or right ventricle (see **Fig. 2**D). Common locations for LGE to appear in sarcoidosis include the basal and mid anteroseptal and inferolateral walls.[21] The presence of LGE detected by CMR is more than twice as sensitive, compared with standardized clinical criteria, for determining whether or not there is cardiac involvement in patients with known sarcoidosis.[22]

Iron overload can result from medical conditions that require frequent blood transfusions. Although LVEF can be reduced in the setting of myocardial iron overload, such a global decrease in systolic function typically manifests in the later stages of advanced disease. Thus, direct assessments of myocardial iron with CMR provide the opportunity to identify iron deposition at an earlier point in the progression of cardiomyopathy and aid in making treatment decisions before the development of severe iron overload or symptomatic HF.[23] CMR is effective because iron deposits alter the appearance of myocardium in specific CMR T1, T2, and T2* sequences. Measurement of T2* has become the most widely used of these sequences because of its superior sensitivity.[24] In fact, the black appearance of iron deposition that is detected by T2* imaging can be reliably quantified using commercial software algorithms.[1]

Unlike other common nonischemic cardiomyopathies, hypertrophic cardiomyopathy (HCM) is known to have a unique structural phenotype that classically involves asymmetric LV wall thickening of the basal interventricular septum. However, among all patients with genotypic disease, wide phenotypic variation exists with respect to structural abnormalities. Nonclassic phenotypes include symmetric, apical, or focal LV hypertrophy involving almost any LV wall segment. Therefore, tissue characterization by CMR can add important complementary information. For instance, LGE is often present in a patchy midwall distribution, particularly at the insertion point of the left and right ventricles and regions of greatest hypertrophy. That said, distribution of LGE in HCM can still be variable and even involve regions of normal wall thickness.[21]

Nonischemic dilated cardiomyopathies are generally recognized to have a typical midwall linear LGE pattern that is commonly located in the ventricular septum (see **Fig. 2**E).[25] It is not yet known what causes this particular pattern of abnormal tissue enhancement on CMR, although this pattern is considered potentially related to the conduction delays often seen in nonischemic dilated cardiomyopathy. In contrast to the more chronic cardiomyopathies, active myocarditis typically demonstrates focal increases in midwall and subepicardial signal on T2-weighted images, signaling the presence of edema in these areas. Farther out from the initial onset of myocarditis, epicardial LGE may be seen in areas of residual fibrosis (see **Fig. 2**F). Using these tissue characteristics, the cause of cardiomyopathy can be derived in many cases and may obviate invasive myocardial biopsy.

FURTHER ASSESSMENTS IN ISCHEMIC CARDIOMYOPATHY

In the setting of stage B HF and known or suspected CAD, CMR can be used to assess for the presence of regional wall motion abnormalities, which are associated with greater burden of coronary artery calcification, even in asymptomatic individuals.[26] Whether wall motion abnormalities are present or absent, several CMR techniques can also be used to comprehensively evaluate for the presence of ischemia and viability.

Ischemia

Guidelines for managing patients with HF suggest that it is reasonable to noninvasively assess for ischemia in patients with HF and known CAD, even in the absence of angina. In this setting, CMR protocols that include stress perfusion imaging can be used to assess for ischemia while offering the advantages of high spatial resolution, excellent image contrast, and no exposure to ionizing radiation. Stress perfusion CMR relies on the principle that differences in myocardial blood flow can be traced using direct visualization of first-pass distribution of gadolinium to regions receiving myocardial blood flow. Gadolinium decreases the T1 time of tissues; thus, T1-weighted sequences run during the first-pass perfusion of gadolinium demonstrate increased enhancement (brighter images) in regions that receive normal perfusion because of the shorter T1 times and, conversely, decreased enhancement (darker images) to regions that have decreased perfusion. These perfusion sequences are run at stress and can be compared with perfusion at rest to assess for a reversible defect suggesting the presence of ischemia.

Stress CMR protocols are commonly performed using a pharmacologic stress agent, given the logistical challenge of performing exercise within a magnetic field. Adenosine, dipyridamole, and regadenoson are vasodilator stress agents that can be administered intravenously to assess for differential hyperemia. A healthy coronary artery allows for approximately 4 times more flow in response to a pharmacologic vasodilator. An artery that has a significant stenosis will be dilated at rest, in the attempt to minimize resistance to intraluminal flow. Because of this phenomenon, a stenosis of greater than 45% results in a reduction in the maximal vasodilatory coronary flow[27] given its baseline vasodilation state. An algorithm that accounts for both the presence of a reversible adenosine-induced perfusion defect and the presence of subendocardial LGE demonstrates 89% sensitivity and 87% specificity in detecting CAD defined as a stenosis of greater than or equal to 70% on invasive cardiac catheterization.[28] Absolute quantification of myocardial perfusion can also be estimated using time-intensity curves to determine myocardial perfusion reserve,[29] which can be used to assess subtle changes in perfusion or to detect 3-vessel disease (balanced ischemia).

Catecholamine stress, via dobutamine administration, increases myocardial oxygen demand and, therefore, can induce a perfusion defect and wall-motion abnormality in vascular territories supplied by vessels with significant stenosis. A dobutamine stress protocol involves starting at a low-dosage infusion (usually 10 μcg/kg/min) and titrating the dosage upwards every 2 to 3 minutes to the target heart rate that is 85% of the age-predicted maximum. Cine images are simultaneously acquired, using a sequence, such as SSFP, with assessments of myocardial wall motion performed at each stage of dobutamine titration. The sensitivity and specificity of a standard dobutamine CMR stress test are 85% and 82%, respectively. Notably, when perfusion imaging is added to wall-motion analyses during the dobutamine stress test, the sensitivity of the test increases to 91%, but specificity is reduced to 70%.[30]

Viability

In the setting of global LV dysfunction and chronic CAD, approximately 25% to 40% of patients have reversible LV dysfunction caused by hibernating myocardium.[31] Hibernating myocardium is viable but it has depressed myocardial contractility at rest because of persistently impaired coronary blood flow.[32] In this setting, function can be partially or completely restored by (1) improving coronary blood flow, (2) providing inotropic stimulation, or (3) reducing oxygen demand.[33] Dysfunctional myocardial territories that have normal blood flow at rest, which may be more common than the classical reduced-flow scenario, demonstrate depressed cardiac function because they undergo recurrent ischemic episodes with stress during repetitive myocardial stunning[31]; in this setting, function can also be improved with revascularization. Diagnosing hibernation as a cause of LV dysfunction is imperative because annual mortality is reduced by 80% with revascularization compared with medical therapy.[34] Conversely, in patients with severe CAD but without evidence of viability, revascularization tends to result in higher rates of death.[34]

Several CMR techniques have been validated regarding their use in the assessment of myocardial viability. A preserved end-diastolic wall thickness (EDWT) of greater than or equal to 5.5 mm at rest has a high sensitivity of 92% but low specificity of 56% for predicting functional recovery following revascularization.[35] Low-dosage dobutamine CMR (5 and 10 μcg/kg/min) can assess viability with improvement in a dysfunctional wall segment by 1 grade (ie, from akinetic to hypokinetic or from hypokinetic to normal), predicting improvement with revascularization 85% of the time.[36] Dobutamine-induced systolic thickening has also been used as a marker for viability, with myocardium deemed viable if greater than or equal to 50% of the segments within an infarcted territory have regions that thicken by greater than or equal to 2 mm despite a resting wall-motion abnormality. This finding has a sensitivity of 89% and a specificity of 94%, suggesting a slightly lower sensitivity but significantly higher specificity than resting EDWT as a marker of recovery following revascularization.[35]

Most CMR centers use the transmural extent of scar as detected by LGE to assess for viability. The high spatial resolution of CMR allows for accurate assessment of the transmural thickness of a scar. CMR-based quantification of LGE is highly correlated with the extent of ex vivo myocyte necrosis in experimental models of MI.[37] In addition, LGE quantitation is highly sensitive for detecting very small areas of subendocardial MI. As little as 2 g of myonecrosis can be detected on LGE sequences in patients who sustain a small creatinine kinase - MB fraction (CK-MB) increase following coronary artery stenting.[38] Accordingly, CMR is a more-sensitive technique for detecting subendocardial infarction than other noninvasive modalities, including positron emission tomography imaging.[39] In a clinical study of 50 patients with CAD and LV dysfunction, the extent of transmural scar assessed by CMR corresponded with the degree of functional recovery following revascularization in a graded fashion.[40] Of the akinetic and dyskinetic segments with no evidence of scar before revascularization, 100% had recovery of function; similar segments with 1% to 25% transmural scar showed 82% recovery of function; segments with 26% to 50% transmural scar had a 45% recovery; segments with 51% to 75% transmural scar had 7% recovery; and similar segments with 76% to 100% scar had 0% recovery. Nonetheless, the limited diagnostic accuracy of LGE in territories with 1% to 75% transmural scar was more recently demonstrated in a study of 29 patients with CAD and LV dysfunction who underwent CMR imaging with both LGE assessment and a low-dosage dobutamine test.[36] The low-dosage dobutamine test was superior to LGE at predicting functional recovery 3 months following revascularization for the subgroup of patients with a 1% to 74% transmural scar. However, there was no significant difference between low-dosage dobutamine stress and LGE in predicting functional recovery in patients without evidence of scar or those with a transmural infarction greater than or equal to 75%.

Additional CMR techniques have been used to assess viability and prognosis following MI. Resting first-pass gadolinium perfusion in combination with LGE an average of 5 days following a reperfused MI had prognostic significance. Territories that hypoenhanced during first-pass perfusion in the setting of a patent epicardial vessel had microvascular obstruction preventing normal flow to the myocardium.[41] Regions that had severe microvascular obstruction do not retain gadolinium and demonstrate no LGE, suggesting no viability and poor functional recovery. T2-weighted imaging for edema within 2 days following a reperfused MI can also assess for viable territories that are at risk if the vessel were to become occluded.[42] Regions of hyperintense T2-weighted imaging indicate myocardial edema and are larger than the infarcted region as demonstrated by LGE. The territories of edema demonstrate partial recovery of systolic function within 2 months of infarction.

RISK STRATIFICATION AND PROGNOSIS

Among all the measures that can be provided by CMR, the LVEF remains the most robust determinant of adverse outcomes in the setting of either ischemic or nonischemic cardiomyopathy. That said, the specific cause of the cardiomyopathy is among the strongest independent determinants of risk, adding prognostic information to LVEF and serving as the primary determinant of outcomes in the setting of a preserved EF. Ischemic cardiomyopathy tends to carry a worse prognosis than nonischemic causes.[43] Among the nonischemic causes, the risk of cardiac events varies widely and also depends largely on the cause of the cardiomyopathy. With the exception of cardiomyopathy caused by HIV, infiltrative cardiomyopathies are associated with the worst prognosis, portending a 4.4-fold greater risk of death relative to idiopathic cardiomyopathy after adjustment for cardiac function. Patients with amyloid and iron overload cardiomyopathy have the worst prognosis among the infiltrative cardiomyopathies, with an associated 7.4-fold and 8.9-fold greater risk of mortality relative to idiopathic cardiomyopathy, respectively.[44] In patients with sarcoidosis, sudden death is a leading cause of mortality, which may represent unrecognized cardiac involvement.[22] Therefore, identifying the underlying cause of cardiomyopathy in all affected patients is critical, especially because some conditions can be improved with targeted interventions. Determining the underlying cause can also provide specific risk stratification for patients who could potentially benefit from ICD placement, as in cases of cardiac sarcoidosis.[45]

Prognosis in Ischemic Cardiomyopathy

The role of CMR as a prognostic tool in patients with CAD has been explored in several studies dating back to Wu and colleagues.[46] In a recent study of 195 patients with a clinical suspicion of CAD, but without a history of MI, the presence of LGE by CMR was associated with an increased risk for major adverse cardiac events (MACE) and cardiac death with hazards of 8.29 and 10.9, respectively ($P<.0001$ for both).[47] This association remained significant after adjusting for clinical, angiographic, and functional variables. In a similar study of patients with diabetes, many of whom had evidence of prior silent MI, presence of LGE was associated with MACE and mortality hazards of 3.71 ($P<.001$) and 3.61 ($P = .007$), respectively, even after adjustment for clinical covariates, electrocardiographic findings, and LV function.[48] For patients with a known prior MI, quantifying the size of the myocardial peri-infarct zone by contrast-enhanced CMR also provides prognostic information. In a study of 144 patients with prior MI, larger areas of peri-infarct tissue conferred higher mortality risk compared with peri-infarct areas below-median area (28% vs 13%, log-rank $P<.01$).[49] Thus, the presence of LGE and size of the peri-infarct zone represent noninvasive CMR parameters that can be used to estimate the risk of adverse outcomes in patients with ischemic cardiomyopathy.

Prognosis in Nonischemic Cardiomyopathies

The role of CMR in risk stratification of patients with nonischemic cardiomyopathy depends on the underlying cause. In a small sample of patients with dilated nonischemic cardiomyopathy referred for an electrophysiology study, the extent of myocardial fibrosis and scar characterized as LGE by CMR has been associated with inducibility of ventricular arrhythmias in these regions.[50] For patients with less-severe disease, there is little evidence overall on prognostic imaging markers, even though these individuals compose most patients with dilated nonischemic cardiomyopathy. In a recent study of 857 patients with and without prior HF, the presence of LGE predicted a 1.3-fold increased risk of cardiac transplantation or death, and results were similar among patients with and without baseline CAD or reduced EF.[51] Although LGE remained significant as a predictor of outcomes in analyses adjusting for prior HF, it is not known how LGE would perform in the subset of patients representing stage B disease without prior HF.

The prognostic value of CMR-based markers of disease has been studied to varying degrees among patients with infiltrative cardiomyopathies. In patients with HCM, the presence of LGE is a frequent finding, with a reported prevalence of 41% among asymptomatic to mildly symptomatic patients[52] and 63% in an unselected sample referred for CMR.[53] In this setting, LGE often reflects regions with decreased myocardial contractility[54] and has been associated with a 7-fold risk of nonsustained ventricular tachycardia on Holter monitoring.[52] With respect to hard endpoints, however, presence versus absence of LGE has limited prognostic value,[53] which may be because of the high prevalence of LGE among all patients with HCM. This finding may also be because the LGE reflects regions of gross focal scarring but not the process of diffuse myocardial fibrosis that is accelerated in HCM. Newer CMR techniques using T1 mapping to assess the distribution of gadolinium between the myocardium and the blood pool can be used to quantify diffuse fibrosis and may prove to have prognostic value in HCM in the future.

The ability of CMR to improve risk stratification in patients with cardiac amyloidosis has also been studied. In a study of 29 patients with known cardiac amyloidosis, the presence of LGE alone was not a significant predictor of death over a mean follow-up of 1.7 years.[55] However, all patients also underwent CMR T1 mapping, similar to the protocol used for patients with HCM, whereby quantification of gadolinium kinetics demonstrated a significant association with mortality risk. In effect, blood gadolinium clearance occurred faster in patients at a higher risk because of the increased interstitial space from amyloid deposition. Additionally, the 2-minute postgadolinium intramyocardial T1 difference between subepicardium and subendocardium predicted mortality with 85% accuracy at a threshold value of 23 milliseconds, indicating that the lower the difference, the worse the prognosis.

CMR-based measures also offer prognostic value in the setting of iron-overload cardiomyopathy. In a study of 652 patients with thalassemia major, cardiac T2* measures predicted cardiac events beyond established predictors, including liver iron and serum ferritin. Lower (<10 milliseconds) compared with higher (>10 milliseconds) cardiac T2* values conferred a markedly increased relative risk for incident HF of 160 (95% confidence interval, 39–653).[24] The area under the receiver-operating characteristic curve (ROC) for predicting HF was significantly greater for cardiac T2* (0.95) than for liver T2* (0.59) or serum ferritin (0.63). The area under the ROC curve for predicting arrhythmia was also significantly greater for cardiac T2* (0.75) than for liver T2* (0.51) or serum ferritin (0.52).[24] These impressive results demonstrate that CMR is a valuable method for determining the prognosis in this group of patients. Accordingly, standard practice for treating iron overload includes adjusting chelation therapy doses based on myocardial T2* levels.[23]

FUTURE DIRECTIONS

Because CMR allows for the ongoing development of different protocols and sequences for imaging the heart, CMR is effectively comprised of multiple imaging techniques that continue to evolve. As such, the potential of CMR to provide additional diagnostic and prognostic information in the evaluation and management of individuals with preclinical cardiac disease continues to grow. On the horizon are technical developments that will likely improve assessments of both structure and function.

With respect to improving characterization of cardiac structure, new CMR techniques have recently been developed to quantify the extent of diffuse myocardial fibrosis present at a given time point. The partition coefficient of gadolinium, the contrast agent that decreases T1 time, can be performed with T1 mapping as performed for the prognostic assessment in patients with HCM and cardiac amyloid. With this technique, decreases in the T1 time of the myocardium reflect increased interstitial space (microfibrosis) and increased gadolinium concentration diffusely throughout the myocardium, with increased gadolinium clearance in the blood pool. Thus, the relative distribution of gadolinium between the blood pool and myocardium can be used to estimate the amount of diffuse fibrosis within the myocardium. When quantified, this relative distribution of gadolinium in the myocardium has been shown to correlate with the presence of fibrosis on surgical biopsies in patients with HCM.[56] Thus, this parameter may prove to be a useful prognostic marker in cardiac amyloid and HCM, in addition to a variety of other disease processes that can lead to abnormal LV remodeling well before the onset of clinical HF and associated outcomes.

With respect to improving assessments of cardiac function, several methods have been developed to allow CMR-based imaging to capture the complexity of myocardial deformation in multiple planes. Of particular interest is myocardial tagging, the technique of noninvasively imprinting tissue tags on the myocardium in a grid or radial pattern to comprehensively track intramyocardial tissue motion and deformation throughout the cardiac cycle (**Fig. 3**). Specifically, CMR myocardial tagging allows for precise measurements of regional strain, ventricular torsion, and segmental synchrony. Alterations in regional and global myocardial tissue deformation, as reflected by measures of systolic and diastolic strain, have been detected by CMR in the setting of cardiovascular risk factors, myocardial ischemia or infarction, nonischemic dilated cardiomyopathy, and HCM, even in patients with a normal EF.[57,58]

Similarly, the extent to which the LV normally undergoes a global twisting motion in systole and untwisting motion (recoil) in diastole, quantified by CMR as measures of torsion, can be impaired in the setting of hypertension and diabetes even when global LV function seems otherwise preserved.[59,60] Likewise, the degree to which myocardial segments contract with decreased synchrony can be quantified using CMR tissue tagging and has also been associated with cardiovascular risk factor burden in the absence of frank LV dysfunction or HF symptoms.[61] Thus, a variety of CMR-based measures now provide the ability to more precisely define phenotypes of subclinical myocardial dysfunction among patients with stage B HF,

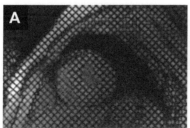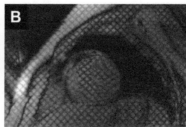

Fig. 3. Myocardial tissue tagging involves using selective radiofrequency bands to noninvasively imprint on the myocardium a grid pattern of tissue markers that track motion and deformation throughout the cardiac cycle. Tissue tagging is shown here in diastole (*A*) and in systole (*B*).

regardless of EF. Such measures can be used to improve identification of individuals with subclinical dysfunction and may also prove to be important for prognosis and risk stratification.

SUMMARY

CMR is a powerful and unique diagnostic tool that can be used to determine the cause and prognosis of patients with asymptomatic cardiomyopathy within a single, reproducible test. CMR also offers the benefit of noninvasively assessing for ischemia and viability in patients with ischemic cardiomyopathy. Given the ongoing development of novel techniques for myocardial tissue characterization and refining phenotypes of subclinical myocardial dysfunction, CMR is likely to continue playing an important role in improving the diagnosis and management of patients at risk for HF.

REFERENCES

1. Sechtem U, Mahrholdt H, Vogelsberg H. Cardiac magnetic resonance in myocardial disease. Heart 2007;93:1520–7.
2. Semelka RC, Tomei E, Wagner S, et al. Interstudy reproducibility of dimensional and functional measurements between cine magnetic resonance studies in the morphologically abnormal left ventricle. Am Heart J 1990;119:1367–73.
3. Daram SR, Cortese CM, Bastani B. Nephrogenic fibrosing dermopathy/nephrogenic systemic fibrosis: report of a new case with literature review. Am J Kidney Dis 2005;46:754–9.
4. Chrysochou C, Power A, Shurrab AE, et al. Low risk for nephrogenic systemic fibrosis in nondialysis patients who have chronic kidney disease and are investigated with gadolinium-enhanced magnetic resonance imaging. Clin J Am Soc Nephrol 2010; 5:484–9.
5. Sadowski EA, Bennett LK, Chan MR, et al. Nephrogenic systemic fibrosis: risk factors and incidence estimation. Radiology 2007;243:148–57.
6. Broome DR, Girguis MS, Baron PW, et al. Gadodiamide-associated nephrogenic systemic fibrosis: why radiologists should be concerned. AJR Am J Roentgenol 2007;188:586–92.
7. Wang TJ, Evans JC, Benjamin EJ, et al. Natural history of asymptomatic left ventricular systolic dysfunction in the community. Circulation 2003; 108:977–82.
8. Bellenger NG, Burgess MI, Ray SG, et al. Comparison of left ventricular ejection fraction and volumes in heart failure by echocardiography, radionuclide ventriculography and cardiovascular magnetic resonance; are they interchangeable? Eur Heart J 2000; 21:1387–96.
9. Teichholz LE, Kreulen T, Herman MV, et al. Problems in echocardiographic volume determinations: echocardiographic-angiographic correlations in the presence of absence of asynergy. Am J Cardiol 1976;37:7–11.
10. Owan TE, Hodge DO, Herges RM, et al. Trends in prevalence and outcome of heart failure with preserved ejection fraction. N Engl J Med 2006; 355:251–9.
11. Paelinck BP, de Roos A, Bax JJ, et al. Feasibility of tissue magnetic resonance imaging: a pilot study in comparison with tissue Doppler imaging and invasive measurement. J Am Coll Cardiol 2005;45: 1109–16.
12. Higgins CB, Sovak M, Schmidt W, et al. Uptake of contrast materials by experimental acute myocardial infarctions: a preliminary report. Invest Radiol 1978; 13:337–9.
13. de Roos A, Doornbos J, van der Wall EE, et al. MR imaging of acute myocardial infarction: value of Gd-DTPA. AJR Am J Roentgenol 1988;150: 531–4.
14. Lima JA, Judd RM, Bazille A, et al. Regional heterogeneity of human myocardial infarcts demonstrated by contrast-enhanced MRI. Potential mechanisms. Circulation 1995;92:1117–25.
15. Rochitte CE, Lima JA, Bluemke DA, et al. Magnitude and time course of microvascular obstruction and tissue injury after acute myocardial infarction. Circulation 1998;98:1006–14.
16. Simonetti OP, Kim RJ, Fieno DS, et al. An improved MR imaging technique for the visualization of myocardial infarction. Radiology 2001;218:215–23.
17. Sievers B, Elliott MD, Hurwitz LM, et al. Rapid detection of myocardial infarction by subsecond, free-breathing delayed contrast-enhancement cardiovascular magnetic resonance. Circulation 2007;115: 236–44.
18. Soriano CJ, Ridocci F, Estornell J, et al. Noninvasive diagnosis of coronary artery disease in patients with heart failure and systolic dysfunction of uncertain etiology, using late gadolinium-enhanced cardiovascular magnetic resonance. J Am Coll Cardiol 2005; 45:743–8.
19. Vogelsberg H, Mahrholdt H, Deluigi CC, et al. Cardiovascular magnetic resonance in clinically suspected cardiac amyloidosis: noninvasive imaging compared to endomyocardial biopsy. J Am Coll Cardiol 2008;51: 1022–30.
20. Rochitte CE, Oliveira PF, Andrade JM, et al. Myocardial delayed enhancement by magnetic resonance imaging in patients with Chagas' disease: a marker of disease severity. J Am Coll Cardiol 2005;46: 1553–8.
21. Karamitsos TD, Francis JM, Myerson S, et al. The role of cardiovascular magnetic resonance imaging in heart failure. J Am Coll Cardiol 2009;54:1407–24.

22. Patel MR, Cawley PJ, Heitner JF, et al. Detection of myocardial damage in patients with sarcoidosis. Circulation 2009;120:1969–77.

23. Brittenham GM. Iron-chelating therapy for transfusional iron overload. N Engl J Med 2011;364:146–56.

24. Kirk P, Roughton M, Porter JB, et al. Cardiac T2* magnetic resonance for prediction of cardiac complications in thalassemia major. Circulation 2009;120:1961–8.

25. Assomull RG, Prasad SK, Lyne J, et al. Cardiovascular magnetic resonance, fibrosis, and prognosis in dilated cardiomyopathy. J Am Coll Cardiol 2006; 48:1977–85.

26. Tsao CW, Gona P, Salton C, et al. Subclinical and clinical correlates of left ventricular wall motion abnormalities in the community. Am J Cardiol 2011;107:949–55.

27. Salerno M, Beller GA. Noninvasive assessment of myocardial perfusion. Circ Cardiovasc Imaging 2009;2:412–24.

28. Klem I, Heitner JF, Shah DJ, et al. Improved detection of coronary artery disease by stress perfusion cardiovascular magnetic resonance with the use of delayed enhancement infarction imaging. J Am Coll Cardiol 2006;47:1630–8.

29. Wilke N, Jerosch-Herold M, Wang Y, et al. Myocardial perfusion reserve: assessment with multisection, quantitative, first-pass MR imaging. Radiology 1997;204:373–84.

30. Gebker R, Jahnke C, Manka R, et al. Additional value of myocardial perfusion imaging during dobutamine stress magnetic resonance for the assessment of coronary artery disease. Circ Cardiovasc Imaging 2008;1:122–30.

31. Bonow RO. Identification of viable myocardium. Circulation 1996;94:2674–80.

32. Rahimtoola SH. Hibernating myocardium has reduced blood flow at rest that increases with low-dose dobutamine. Circulation 1996;94:3055–61.

33. Wijns W, Vatner SF, Camici PG. Hibernating myocardium. N Engl J Med 1998;339:173–81.

34. Allman KC, Shaw LJ, Hachamovitch R, et al. Myocardial viability testing and impact of revascularization on prognosis in patients with coronary artery disease and left ventricular dysfunction: a meta-analysis. J Am Coll Cardiol 2002;39:1151–8.

35. Baer FM, Theissen P, Schneider CA, et al. Dobutamine magnetic resonance imaging predicts contractile recovery of chronically dysfunctional myocardium after successful revascularization. J Am Coll Cardiol 1998;31:1040–8.

36. Wellnhofer E, Olariu A, Klein C, et al. Magnetic resonance low-dose dobutamine test is superior to SCAR quantification for the prediction of functional recovery. Circulation 2004;109:2172–4.

37. Kim RJ, Fieno DS, Parrish TB, et al. Relationship of MRI delayed contrast enhancement to irreversible injury, infarct age, and contractile function. Circulation 1999;100:1992–2002.

38. Ricciardi MJ, Wu E, Davidson CJ, et al. Visualization of discrete microinfarction after percutaneous coronary intervention associated with mild creatine kinase-MB elevation. Circulation 2001;103:2780–3.

39. Klein C, Nekolla SG, Bengel FM, et al. Assessment of myocardial viability with contrast-enhanced magnetic resonance imaging: comparison with positron emission tomography. Circulation 2002;105: 162–7.

40. Kim RJ, Wu E, Rafael A, et al. The use of contrast-enhanced magnetic resonance imaging to identify reversible myocardial dysfunction. N Engl J Med 2000;343:1445–53.

41. Rogers WJ Jr, Kramer CM, Geskin G, et al. Early contrast-enhanced MRI predicts late functional recovery after reperfused myocardial infarction. Circulation 1999;99:744–50.

42. Aletras AH, Tilak GS, Natanzon A, et al. Retrospective determination of the area at risk for reperfused acute myocardial infarction with T2-weighted cardiac magnetic resonance imaging: histopathological and displacement encoding with stimulated echoes (DENSE) functional validations. Circulation 2006;113:1865–70.

43. Bart BA, Shaw LK, McCants CB Jr, et al. Clinical determinants of mortality in patients with angiographically diagnosed ischemic or nonischemic cardiomyopathy. J Am Coll Cardiol 1997;30:1002–8.

44. Felker GM, Thompson RE, Hare JM, et al. Underlying causes and long-term survival in patients with initially unexplained cardiomyopathy. N Engl J Med 2000;342:1077–84.

45. Epstein AE, DiMarco JP, Ellenbogen KA, et al. ACC/AHA/HRS 2008 guidelines for device-based therapy of cardiac rhythm abnormalities: a report of the American College of Cardiology/American Heart Association Task Force on Practice Guidelines (Writing Committee to Revise the ACC/AHA/NASPE 2002 Guideline Update for Implantation of Cardiac Pacemakers and Antiarrhythmia Devices) developed in collaboration with the American Association for Thoracic Surgery and Society of Thoracic Surgeons. J Am Coll Cardiol 2008;51:e1–62.

46. Wu KC, Kim RJ, Bluemke DA, et al. Quantification and time course of microvascular obstruction by contrast-enhanced echocardiography and magnetic resonance imaging following acute myocardial infarction and reperfusion. J Am Coll Cardiol 1998; 32:1756–64.

47. Kwong RY, Chan AK, Brown KA, et al. Impact of unrecognized myocardial scar detected by cardiac magnetic resonance imaging on event-free survival in patients presenting with signs or symptoms of coronary artery disease. Circulation 2006;113: 2733–43.

48. Kwong RY, Sattar H, Wu H, et al. Incidence and prognostic implication of unrecognized myocardial scar characterized by cardiac magnetic resonance in diabetic patients without clinical evidence of myocardial infarction. Circulation 2008;118: 1011–20.

49. Yan AT, Shayne AJ, Brown KA, et al. Characterization of the peri-infarct zone by contrast-enhanced cardiac magnetic resonance imaging is a powerful predictor of post-myocardial infarction mortality. Circulation 2006;114:32–9.

50. Nazarian S, Bluemke DA, Lardo AC, et al. Magnetic resonance assessment of the substrate for inducible ventricular tachycardia in nonischemic cardiomyopathy. Circulation 2005;112:2821–5.

51. Cheong BY, Muthupillai R, Wilson JM, et al. Prognostic significance of delayed-enhancement magnetic resonance imaging: survival of 857 patients with and without left ventricular dysfunction. Circulation 2009;120:2069–76.

52. Adabag AS, Maron BJ, Appelbaum E, et al. Occurrence and frequency of arrhythmias in hypertrophic cardiomyopathy in relation to delayed enhancement on cardiovascular magnetic resonance. J Am Coll Cardiol 2008;51:1369–74.

53. O'Hanlon R, Grasso A, Roughton M, et al. Prognostic significance of myocardial fibrosis in hypertrophic cardiomyopathy. J Am Coll Cardiol 2010; 56:867–74.

54. Ghio S, Revera M, Mori F, et al. Regional abnormalities of myocardial deformation in patients with hypertrophic cardiomyopathy: correlations with delayed enhancement in cardiac magnetic resonance. Eur J Heart Fail 2009;11:952–7.

55. Maceira AM, Prasad SK, Hawkins PN, et al. Cardiovascular magnetic resonance and prognosis in cardiac amyloidosis. J Cardiovasc Magn Reson 2008;10:54.

56. Flett AS, Hayward MP, Ashworth MT, et al. Equilibrium contrast cardiovascular magnetic resonance for the measurement of diffuse myocardial fibrosis: preliminary validation in humans. Circulation 2010; 122:138–44.

57. Shehata ML, Cheng S, Osman NF, et al. Myocardial tissue tagging with cardiovascular magnetic resonance. J Cardiovasc Magn Reson 2009;11:55.

58. Azevedo CF, Cheng S, Lima JA. Cardiac imaging to identify patients at risk for developing heart failure after myocardial infarction. Curr Heart Fail Rep 2005;2:183–8.

59. Chung J, Abraszewski P, Yu X, et al. Paradoxical increase in ventricular torsion and systolic torsion rate in type I diabetic patients under tight glycemic control. J Am Coll Cardiol 2006;47:384–90.

60. Takeuchi M, Otsuji Y, Lang RM. Evaluation of left ventricular function using left ventricular twist and torsion parameters. Curr Cardiol Rep 2009;11: 225–30.

61. Rosen BD, Fernandes VR, Nasir K, et al. Age, increased left ventricular mass, and lower regional myocardial perfusion are related to greater extent of myocardial dyssynchrony in asymptomatic individuals: the multi-ethnic study of atherosclerosis. Circulation 2009;120:859–66.

Radionuclide Imaging in Stage B Heart Failure

Rajesh Janardhanan, MD, MRCP, George A. Beller, MD*

KEYWORDS

- Radionuclide imaging • Stage B heart failure
- Asymptomatic left ventricular dysfunction
- Ischemic cardiomyopathy • Viability
- Single-photon emission computed tomography
- Positron emission tomography

Despite significant advances in the prevention and treatment of cardiovascular disease in the past 2 decades, the incidence and prevalence of chronic heart failure have been increasing. Heart failure (HF) affects approximately 5 million individuals in the United States, but remains a poorly understood and inadequately treated condition.[1,2]

Stage B heart failure,[3] as defined by the American College of Cardiology (ACC)/American Heart Association (AHA) guidelines, includes patients with structural heart disease but no current or prior symptoms of HF. Once a patient experiences symptoms of HF, they advance to stage C even if they later become asymptomatic. The current guidelines stipulate that patients may only move forward through the stages and not regress. The guidelines of the ACC and the AHA have emphasized the importance of the detection of early disease in patients at risk (stage A) and those with asymptomatic left ventricular dysfunction (ALVD) or stage B.[4]

Radionuclide imaging appears to be well suited for the evaluation of patients with Stage B HF. This article discusses currently available radionuclide techniques in the diagnostic and prognostic evaluation of patients with chronic HF with a focus on stage B/asymptomatic left ventricular (LV) dysfunction.

STAGE B HEART FAILURE: IMPORTANCE OF RECOGNITION

The number of patients with chronic HF and impaired systolic function in stage B is estimated to be 4 times greater than in stages C and D combined.[5] In a community-based study, Wang and colleagues[6] observed that more than half of all patients with impaired systolic function were asymptomatic. These patients remain at risk for significant morbidity and mortality and the subsequent development of symptomatic HF. Despite the high risk associated with ALVD, these patients often go undetected and untreated. Patients with ALVD who are not admitted to the hospital are undoubtedly even less likely to be recognized and treated.

It is important to recognize that the largest proportion of patients with stage B HF evaluated in clinical trials have had an ischemic origin, from either a recognized myocardial infarction (MI) or subclinical myocardial necrosis, often exacerbated by hypertension and/or diabetes mellitus.[3] Ischemia in the form of angina or MI is often the trigger to evaluate an otherwise asymptomatic patient and discover the LV dysfunction. In addition, a smaller but still sizable number of patients with ALVD present with a nonischemic cause, including those with hypertensive or valvular heart

The authors have nothing to disclose.
Division of Cardiology, University of Virginia Health System, Box 800158, Charlottesville, VA 22908, USA
* Corresponding author.
E-mail address: gbeller@virginia.edu

Heart Failure Clin 8 (2012) 191–206
doi:10.1016/j.hfc.2011.11.004

disease, cardiotoxin exposure, postviral infection/myocarditis, nonischemic dilated cardiomyopathy, and familial dilated cardiomyopathy.

It is possible, of course, that many patients with ALVD minimize or deny their symptoms, despite demonstrable exercise intolerance. The onset of HF symptoms is gradual and may not be appreciated or acknowledged by patients. Such patients may remain apparently symptom-free by unconsciously reducing activity levels to compensate for worsening exertional symptoms. Therefore, clinicians may need objective testing, such as imaging, including formal exercise testing, to truly differentiate stage B patients from those with stage C, which makes the identification of stage B patients in epidemiologic or treatment trials more challenging.[3]

ROLE OF RADIONUCLIDE IMAGING IN STAGE B HEART FAILURE
Assessment of Left Ventricular Dysfunction

Although 2-dimensional echocardiography is most widely used to evaluate LV systolic function, radionuclide techniques are well validated for this application. Among the available radionuclide techniques, equilibrium radionuclide angiocardiography (ERNA) or radionuclide ventriculography (RVG) has been traditionally used to determine LV systolic and diastolic function. Serial LV ejection fraction (LVEF) data are particularly important in patients undergoing chemotherapy for cancer, known cardiomyopathies, and after undergoing transplantation.

ERNA has been largely supplanted by gated single-photon emission computed tomography (SPECT) imaging, which is extensively used for the assessment of myocardial perfusion and provides simultaneous information on global and regional LV systolic function. Assessment of LVEF by gated SPECT imaging has been validated against other established imaging modalities, including echocardiography, radionuclide ventriculography, and newer techniques with high spatial resolution such as magnetic resonance imaging, with excellent correlation.[7] Gated SPECT in Stage B HF offers comprehensive evaluation of LV systolic function and myocardial perfusion. Right ventricular dysfunction can also be identified by ERNA and gated SPECT.

Compared with 2-dimensional echocardiography, a significant advantage of gated SPECT estimation of LV systolic function is its fully automated application, resulting in high reproducibility. Studies indicate that the variability in serial estimations of LVEF from gated rest ^{99m}Tc-SPECT scans is only approximately $\pm 5\%$.[8,9] Hence the

technique may be suitable for serial assessment of LVEF, as in patients undergoing chemotherapy with potential cardiotoxic agents.

Radionuclide Imaging in Ischemic Cardiomyopathy

The National Health and Nutrition Evaluation Survey (NHANES) I Epidemiologic Follow-up Study of more than 13,000 men and women without HF at baseline found that after an average of 19 years, more than 60% of all HF cases were attributable to coronary artery disease (CAD).[10] Nevertheless, CAD may still be underestimated as the cause of HF, because ischemic cardiomyopathy (ICM) may be present without a history of MI, angina, or other distinct ischemic events.[2] In the Studies of Left Ventricular Dysfunction (SOLVD) prevention trial of 4228 patients with ALVD, 83% had a history of ischemic CAD.[11]

Identification of patients with ALVD from underlying significant CAD represents an important subset of patients in whom myocardial revascularization could potentially prevent progression to overt HF. Current practice guidelines mandate coronary angiography in HF patients with angina.[4] However, up to 60% of patients with ischemic LV dysfunction do not have angina,[12] and the guidelines do not offer firm recommendations for the optimal initial evaluation strategy of these patients.[4,13]

Diagnosis of CAD in heart failure
SPECT imaging to diagnosing CAD in HF Only a scant amount of available literature exists on radionuclide imaging pertaining specifically to Stage B HF. However, the role of myocardial perfusion imaging (MPI) to diagnose CAD noninvasively in patients with HF in general has been investigated.[14]

Many of these studies predated contemporary MPI methodology, for example, using nongated, planar thallium-201 (^{201}Tl) scintigraphy, and yet showed a near perfect sensitivity and negative predictive value (NPV) **(Table 1)**, but modest specificity and positive predictive value.[14]

Gated technetium-99m (^{99m}Tc)-sestamibi SPECT MPI incorporating information on both perfusion and regional LV function demonstrated a high sensitivity of 94% but specificity of only 45%.[15] Thus, these studies performed in patients with chronic HF (although not specifically limited to stage B HF) suggest that MPI may be used to exclude significant CAD with a high degree of accuracy, but because of the poor specificity of the technique, many HF patients without CAD will undergo coronary angiography based on falsely positive MPI results.

Table 1
Clinical studies of myocardial perfusion imaging in chronic heart failure

Author	Technique	Negative Predictive Value (%)	Positive Predictive Value (%)
Bulkley (1977)	Tl-201	100	72
Dunn (1982)	Tl-201	100	40
Saltissi (1981)	Tl-201	100	65
Eichorn (1988)	Tl-201	100	71
Tauberg (1993)	Tl-201	100	61
Chikamori (1992)	Tl-201	100	65

Abbreviation: Tl, thallium.
Data from Udelson JE, Shafer CD, Carrio I. Radionuclide imaging in heart failure: assessing etiology and outcomes and implications for management. J Nucl Cardiol 2002;9(Suppl 5):40S–52S.

The IMAGING in Heart Failure study,[16] comprising 201 patients hospitalized for their first episode of HF, underwent rest/stress gated ^{99m}Tc-sestamibi SPECT as an initial investigative strategy during their index hospitalization. SPECT performance characteristics revealed an excellent NPV of 96% for extensive CAD (ie, normal perfusion or small defect size suggesting nonischemic cardiomyopathy). Normal perfusion was noted in 41%. Of those with abnormal perfusion, fixed defects due to prior MI were common. By multivariate analysis, the extent of perfusion abnormality and advancing age predicted the presence of extensive CAD. In addition, 36% of patients had preserved LV systolic function. Even though these patients had acute HF, SPECT MPI would surely be useful in identifying extensive CAD as the cause of ALVD.

Caution needs to be exercised in the use of stress SPECT for differentiating ischemic from nonischemic cardiomyopathy. Considerable overlap of scar patterns was seen between 14 patients with ICM and 15 patients with nonischemic dilated cardiomyopathy with an LVEF of less than 40% who underwent ^{201}Tl-SPECT.[17] Patients with ICM had a higher summed stress defect score (27.9 ± 9.4 vs 20.6 ± 8.9; P = .04) and more moderate or severe perfusion defect segments on stress scans (7.2 ± 2.0 vs 4.5 ± 2.6; P = .004) than did patients with nonischemic dilated cardiomyopathy. However, as noted, considerable overlap between the groups

was observed. Yet moderate or severe defects post stress in at least 7 of the 17 segments were seen in 71% of patients with ICM compared with 20% in those with nonischemic cardiomyopathy (P = .016).

False-positive SPECT MPI results for CAD in HF The predominant cause of false positivity for CAD is soft-tissue attenuation, although pathophysiologic phenomena such as myocardial fibrosis and endothelial dysfunction resulting in reduced coronary reserve produce abnormal MPI in some patients with unobstructed epicardial coronary arteries.[18,19]

Although quantitative attenuation-correction techniques have been shown in clinical trials to improve diagnostic specificity of SPECT MPI, this approach has not been tested specifically in patients with HF.[20] Given the propensity of attenuation artifacts in patients with a dilated left ventricle, attenuation correction is likely to favorably impact specificity in this population. It is also possible that MPI combined with computed tomography (CT) could obviate in the future the need for invasive coronary angiography, because of the added high NPV of normal anatomic CT angiography.[21–23]

Positron emission tomography MPI in diagnosing CAD in HF Positron emission tomography (PET) MPI offers unique possibilities for quantification of basal and hyperemic regional myocardial perfusion, which is useful in patients with diffuse CAD or balanced reduction in perfusion due to severe 3-vessel disease,[24] for whom the relative assessment of myocardial perfusion by SPECT may fail in uncovering true perfusion changes.

Assessment of viability, ischemia, and myocardial hibernation in ICM
Noninvasive investigation of the presence and extent of myocardial viability and ischemia is an important component of the diagnostic evaluation of all patients with LV dysfunction and known CAD.

SPECT imaging In patients with ischemic LV dysfunction, the assessment of myocardial viability is a critical step in management planning. On one hand, patients with severe LV systolic dysfunction undergoing coronary bypass grafting are at high risk for perioperative mortality.[25] On the other hand, the presence of significant amounts of residual myocardial viability portends the potential for improvement in symptoms,[26–28] regional LV function,[29,30] global LV function,[31,32] and prognosis[33,34] following coronary revascularization (**Fig. 1**). It must be noted that although the use of functional recovery is a convenient standard

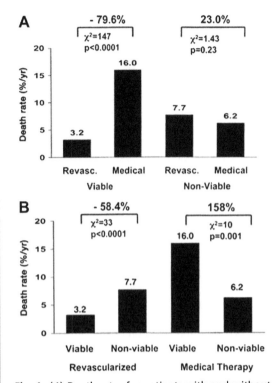

Fig. 1. (A) Death rates for patients with and without myocardial viability treated by revascularization or medical therapy. (B) Same data as in a with comparisons based on treatment strategy in patients with and without viability. (Reproduced from Allman KC, Shaw LJ, Hachamovitch R, et al. Myocardial viability testing and impact of revascularization on prognosis in patients with coronary artery disease and left ventricular dysfunction: a meta-analysis. J Am Coll Cardiol 2002;39(7):1151–8; with permission.)

for viability studies it may not capture the full benefit of revascularization, which may confer other important benefits such as attenuation of progressive remodeling, prevention of functional mitral regurgitation, and prevention of arrhythmia independently of functional recovery.[35–37] LV function may also continue to improve for several months following revascularization, so a single assessment, if not timed appropriately, may underestimate the full extent of functional recovery.[36] Finally, resting regional function is primarily determined by endocardial thickening, which is unlikely to improve in patients who have suffered a subendocardial MI despite preserved myocardial viability.[38–40] A more important criterion for assessing the usefulness of noninvasive viability testing should be whether it can drive therapeutic decisions that ultimately improve patient outcome.

Both ^{201}Tl-labeled (**Fig. 2**) and ^{99m}Tc-labeled myocardial perfusion tracers (**Fig. 3**) are used in

combination with SPECT for clinical evaluation of myocardial viability (**Fig. 4**).[41,42] Different protocols for the assessment of myocardial viability by ^{201}Tl imaging are available; the most frequently used being stress-redistribution-reinjection and rest-redistribution. The first provides information on both stress-inducible ischemia and viability whereas the latter provides information only on viability.

On ^{201}Tl imaging, dysfunctional but viable myocardium can show any of these[42]: (1) normal ^{201}Tl uptake (normal perfusion) at stress, (2) a perfusion defect at stress with redistribution on the 3- to 4-hour delayed images, (3) perfusion defects at stress, without redistribution at 3- to 4-hour delayed imaging (fixed defects), with fill-in after reinjection or delayed rest images, and (4) tracer uptake greater than 50% on the redistribution/reinjection images, or the delayed rest images.

The property of redistribution confers an advantage to ^{201}Tl compared with ^{99m}Tc agents for viability assessment in dysfunctional myocardial segments supplied by a critically stenosed coronary artery. The continued uptake of ^{201}Tl over time results in higher tracer uptake on the delayed scan than on the early scan, thus signaling the presence of viable myocardium.[43,44] However, when used with nitrate enhancement and quantitative interpretation, ^{99m}Tc-sestamibi SPECT has comparable accuracy for viability assessment.[45,46]

With electrocardiogram-gated SPECT the simultaneous assessment of perfusion and wall motion is possible, which improves sensitivity to detect viable myocardium, but may also lower specificity. Administration of nitrates before tracer injection may further improve diagnostic accuracy, probably because nitrates enhance myocardial perfusion (and tracer uptake) in myocardial regions related to a severely stenosed coronary artery, presumably by enhancing collateral blood flow.

Clinical studies suggest that residual myocardial viability is prevalent among patients with ischemic LV dysfunction.[47,48] For example, in the CHRISTMAS trial of 489 patients with chronic HF due to ischemic LV dysfunction (LVEF 29% ± 11%), 79% had viable myocardium demonstrated by ^{99m}Tc-sestamibi SPECT imaging.[48] It must be noted that viability exists as a continuum, ranging from patients with extensive scar tissue and minimal residual viability, to those with minimal scar tissue and predominantly viable but dysfunctional myocardium caused by varying combinations of hibernating and repetitive stunning.[49,50] Patient outcome is dependent on not only the presence but also the extent of viability, and a critical threshold mass of viable myocardium may be

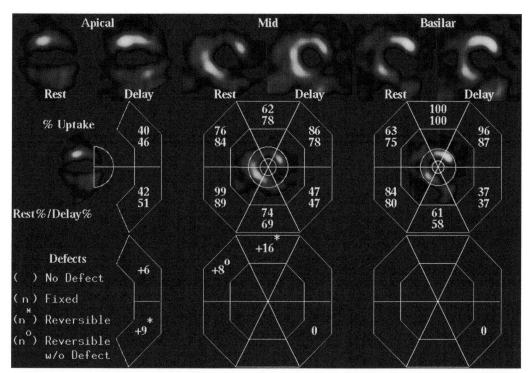

Fig. 2. [201]Tl rest and delayed quantitative SPECT images in a patient with left ventricular dysfunction from ischemic cardiomyopathy, demonstrating rest-redistribution in the anterior wall and septum suggesting viability and a severe stenosis of the left anterior descending artery, and a severe fixed defect in the inferolateral wall suggesting absence of viability in that territory. The numbers in the diagrams below the SPECT images show percent uptake of the tracer on initial rest images (Rest; top numbers) and the 3-hour delayed images (Delay; bottom numbers) related to the area of highest uptake, which is normalized at 100%. The last set of diagrams at the bottom relate to the change in segmental defect magnitude between the 2 images.

necessary for functional recovery and prognostic benefit to occur from revascularization.[51] Therefore, while several clinical and laboratory parameters, including anginal symptoms, absence of Q waves on the electrocardiogram, and absence of thinning and akinesis on echocardiography, indicate the presence of some viability, a systematic assessment of the degree and extent of viability is often indicated for management planning and prognostication.

PET imaging PET has been considered for many years as the gold standard for assessment of myocardial viability using metabolic tracers. The advantage of PET is the ability to label naturally occurring elements in the body such as carbon, oxygen, and nitrogen. For assessment of myocardial perfusion, oxygen-15 water, nitrogen-13 ammonia (NH_3), and rubidium-82 chloride can be used. Currently available tracers for the assessment of myocardial metabolism are the glucose analogue fluorine-18 fluorodeoxyglucose (FDG) and, less commonly, carbon-11 acetate. NH_3/FDG-PET or rubidium-82/FDG-

PET are the most common combinations for the detection of hibernation in clinical practice (see **Fig. 4**).

Dysfunctional myocardial segments with higher FDG uptake compared with that of NH_3 or rubidium-82 (mismatch between and perfusion and metabolism) represent hibernating myocardium (**Fig. 5**), while reduction on both perfusion and metabolism suggests the presence of scarring. In cases of myocardial stunning, perfusion is normal or almost normal while the FDG uptake is variable. The sensitivity and specificity of FDG-PET for segmental recovery of hibernating myocardium after revascularization are 89% and 57%, respectively, with positive and NPVs of 73% and 90%, respectively.[52] The greatest improvement in HF symptoms after revascularization occurs in patients with the largest PET mismatch defects (**Fig. 6**).[26]

Comparing radionuclide methods of viability testing Radionuclide techniques used for viability assessment are based on the demonstration of preserved myocyte metabolism (FDG-PET) or

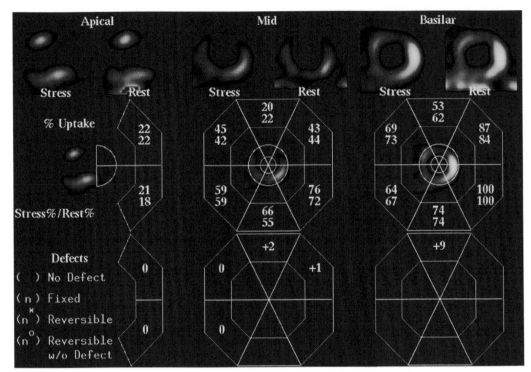

Fig. 3. Stress and resting ^{99m}Tc-sestamibi SPECT images in a patient with left ventricular dysfunction from a prior anterior wall myocardial infarction, showing a severe large anterior and apical fixed defect suggesting absence of viability in that vascular territory. The quantitative analysis shows that the tracer uptake is reduced to 22% of the highest uptake in the mid anterior wall, indicating very poor viability. The basal slices show some inducible anterior ischemia, which is mild (9% defect) reversibility.

cellular integrity (SPECT with ^{201}Tl or ^{99m}Tc ligands). The use of PET and SPECT for viability assessment is supported by a substantial body of literature, with SPECT having the advantages of wider availability and relative ease of use, and PET having a slightly higher overall accuracy.[29] The high-energy photons released from the annihilation of positrons with PET confer a spatial resolution superior to SPECT. Furthermore, combination with attenuation correction allows quantitative analysis of regional myocardial blood flow and metabolism using PET imaging.

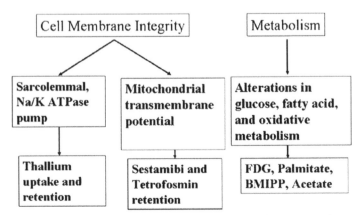

Fig. 4. Schematic physiologic basis for assessing myocardial viability with nuclear radiotracers. ATP, adenosine triphosphate; BMIPP, 15-(p-iodophenyl)-3-(R,S) methlypentadecanoic acid; FDG, fluorodeoxyglucose. (*Reproduced from* Arrighi JA, Dilsizian V. Nuclear probes for assessing myocardial viability in heart failure. Heart Fail Clin 2006;2(2):129–43; with permission.)

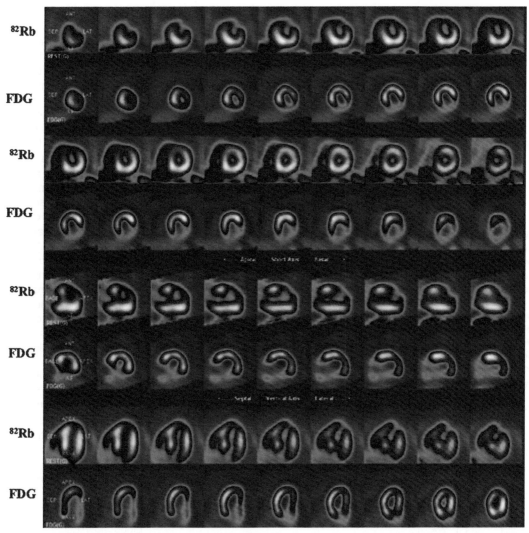

Fig. 5. Upregulation of glucose , evidenced by increased ^{18}F-fluorodeoxyglucose (FDG) uptake in areas of hypo-perfused myocardium (ie, PET mismatch) may identify a high-risk population for cardiac complications and serve as a marker for clinical instability. (*Reproduced from* Marwick TH, Schwaiger M. The future of cardiovascular imaging in the diagnosis and management of heart failure, part 2: clinical applications. Circ Cardiovasc Imaging 2008;1(2):162–70; with permission.)

The major disadvantages of PET are its limited availability and cost. For instance, although oxygen-15 water has a myocardial extraction fraction of virtually 100% and is hence an excellent tracer of myocardial perfusion, it must be manufactured using an on-site cyclotron because of its very short half-life. Nitrogen-13 NH_3 is also difficult to access unless there is on-site cyclotron. Thus, in clinical practice rubidium-82 is the most widely used PET radiotracer for the assessment of myocardial perfusion. A rubidium generator lasts for 1 month but it is relatively expensive. To overcome the limitations related to PET perfusion tracers, some centers have adopted a hybrid (SPECT/PET) approach combining FDG-PET with a SPECT perfusion tracer such as ^{201}Tl or ^{99m}Tc. Although conceptually this is an interesting combination,[53] there are technical issues regarding the comparison of PET and SPECT images.

Radionuclide imaging in evaluation of prognosis in ICM

The composite of currently available data in the literature suggests that HF patients with extensive myocardial perfusion abnormalities are likely to have etiologically related and prognostically significant CAD, and are therefore likely to benefit from coronary revascularization, whereas patients with normal MPI are unlikely to have prognostically significant CAD.

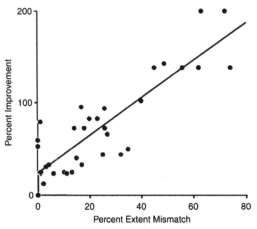

Fig. 6. Scatter plot showing the relation between the anatomic extent of blood flow-metabolism PET mismatch pattern, expressed as percent of the left ventricle, and the change in functional status after coronary artery bypass grafting, expressed as percent improvement in heart failure from baseline. The greatest improvement in symptoms of heart failure occurs in patients with the largest PET mismatch defects. (*Adapted from* Di Carli MF, Asgarzadie F, Schelbert HR, et al. Quantitative relation between myocardial viability and improvement in heart failure symptoms after revascularization in patients with ischemic cardiomyopathy. Circulation 1995;92(12): 3436–44; with permission.)

Infarct size can be accurately estimated by SPECT imaging and is closely associated with subsequent LVEF, LV end-systolic volume, and LV remodeling after acute MI (**Fig. 7**). Resting SPECT can be used to distinguish myocardial

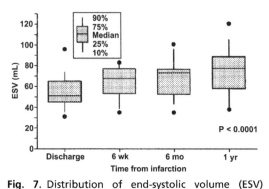

Fig. 7. Distribution of end-systolic volume (ESV) through 4 points in time after acute infarction. Box plots represent median value and 25th and 75th percentiles with the 10th and 90th percentiles; outliers are plotted separately (*circles*). There was a significant increase in ESV over 1 year (P<.0001). (*Adapted from* Chareonthaitawee P, Christian TF, Hirose K, et al. Relation of initial infarct size to extent of left ventricular remodeling in the year after acute myocardial infarction. J Am Coll Cardiol 1995;25(3): 567–73; with permission.).

stunning from irreversible myocardial injury as the cause of ALVD after reperfusion. It is the mismatch between infarct size and ventricular function after reperfusion therapy that identifies postperfusion stunning (ie, small infarct size with more extensive regional dysfunction and intact perfusion).[54–56]

The clinical relevance of detecting patients with viable, hibernating myocardium has become apparent because many such patients have the potential for substantial improvement in regional and global LV function after myocardial revascularization.[36,51,57,58] Although improvement of regional and global LV function after revascularization is important, the most important goal of revascularizing dysfunctional but viable myocardium is improvement of long-term prognosis.[42] It is assumed that the improvement in LVEF translates into better outcome.[59] The data from small nonrandomized series suggest that this improvement in ventricular function after revascularization translates into an improvement in HF symptoms and enhanced survival.[26,60–62]

Although viability testing is somewhat limited by the lack of randomized control studies, a meta-analysis by Allman and colleagues[33] of 24 studies of viability testing with MPI or dobutamine echocardiography that reported on survival after coronary revascularization provides important insights. In patients with predominantly viable myocardium, follow-up on medical therapy was associated with a 16% annual mortality. Similar patients who were revascularized experienced an annual mortality of only 3.2%, that is, an 80% reduction in mortality. By contrast, the choice of medical therapy or revascularization had no significant impact on annual mortality (7.7% vs 6.2%, respectively) in patients with predominantly nonviable myocardium. Despite the known limitations of a meta-analysis, these data provide a strong signal that the presence of residual myocardial viability in patients with LV systolic dysfunction is a marker of very high risk without revascularization.

When compared with other imaging modalities for viability assessment, radionuclide techniques have comparable predictive accuracy for functional recovery.[29] Comparative studies also indicate that slight differences in sensitivity and specificity among these modalities may not affect management decision making in a clinically meaningful way.[63] Furthermore, other information that can be derived from PET and SPECT imaging, such as the degree of remodeling, may interact with the amount of residual viability to determine outcome after revascularization.[64]

Compared with the large volume of data available on the prognostic utility of myocardial perfusion scanning (MPS) in unselected patients referred for stress testing and several subgroups therein, there is only a relatively scant amount of literature pertaining specifically to the use of MPS to determine prognosis in patients with HF.[65] In one of the very few prospectively conducted studies of the prognostic utility of MPS in the HF population, Candell-Riera and colleagues[66] analyzed the predictive variables for prognosis in ICM in patients with CAD and LVEF of 40% or less consecutively studied with gated SPECT with an average follow-up of over 2 years. Although this study did not exclusively study patients with stage B HF, the data are pertinent to that population.

In this study, 167 patients with ICM consecutively underwent rest myocardial perfusion-gated SPECT. The mortality rate over this relatively short period of follow-up was substantial: 22% (36/167) all-cause mortality, of which 17% (29/167) were cardiac deaths. As expected, the majority of deaths in this population were from progressive HF (23), and most of the remainder were sudden cardiac deaths. On univariable analysis, patients who died of cardiac causes were older, less often able to undergo exercise testing, and had a greater prevalence of myocardial viability. Independent predictors of cardiac mortality in rest-gated SPECT were the positive criteria for myocardial viability ($P = .027$; hazard risk, 5.1; 95% confidence interval, 1.2–21.4).

In addition, stress SPECT was performed on 137 of these patients who did not have overt HF. Among these patients who were able to undergo exercise testing the survivors had greater exercise intensity and duration, with a lower prevalence of combined ischemia and viability, but not ischemia alone. Numerous other clinical and electrocardiographic criteria, and notably all coronary angiographic criteria, were similar between these groups. In a multivariable model that included the entire study group of 167 patients, myocardial viability and the inability to exercise were associated with cardiac death. In patients able to exercise, exercise intensity of less than 75 W, exercise duration of 5 minutes or less (cutoffs determined by receiver-operating characteristic curve analysis), myocardial viability and ischemia were associated with cardiac death. The addition of the exercise MPS to the gated MPS variables significantly improved the χ^2 values of the model, thus establishing incremental prognostic value. It is worth emphasizing once again that coronary angiography variables in this cohort of patients did not significantly modify the prognostic value of noninvasive testing.

This incremental prognostic value created by the addition of exercise MPS to the gated MPS could be potentially extrapolated to patients with stage B HF, who are more likely to be able to exercise than patients with symptomatic HF.

Added prognostic value of gated SPECT

Gated SPECT significantly increases the prognostic value of clinical variables for cardiac mortality and nonfatal MI in patients with chronic or suspected ischemic heart disease.[67] The sum of prognostic exercise variables and myocardial perfusion abnormalities provides more powerful prognostic information than clinical variables alone. In patients with ICM, Candell-Riera and colleagues[66] noted that irrespective of the treatment strategy adopted, scintigraphic viability criteria on gated SPECT significantly correlated with greater cardiac mortality, becoming even more significant when associated with scintigraphic criteria of ischemia. Eighty-seven percent of cardiac deaths were in patients who had criteria for viability and ischemia in gated myocardial perfusion SPECT.[66]

Another variable of unquestionable prognostic value in patients with chronic ischemic heart disease, or following an acute MI, is LVEF. Curtis and colleagues[68] studied 7788 patients with stable HF, and observed that there were no significant differences in mortality when patients with LVEF between 45% and 55% were compared with patients whose values exceeded 55%. However, when LVEF was less than 45% there was an inverse relationship between LVEF and mortality.

Radionuclide Imaging in Nonischemic Cardiomyopathy

The literature on radionuclide imaging in nonischemic cardiomyopathy is limited. In patients with severe LV dysfunction but limited-extent CAD (eg, single-vessel disease), the underlying pathophysiology is unlikely to be ischemic LV dysfunction but rather cardiomyopathy of other etiology coexisting with minor CAD. This distinction between patients with LV dysfunction resulting from extensive CAD and those with nonischemic LV dysfunction coexisting with limited-extent CAD is prognostically important (**Fig. 8**).[69] In certain situations, PET imaging may be helpful to identify nonischemic causes of LV dysfunction (**Fig. 9**).

Emerging Role of Nuclear Cardiology

Nuclear techniques for molecular imaging of the myocardium such as those involved in the processes of myocardial perfusion, metabolism and viability, cellular injury, dyssynchrony, interstitial dysregulation, and neurohormonal receptor function may facilitate better clinical outcomes

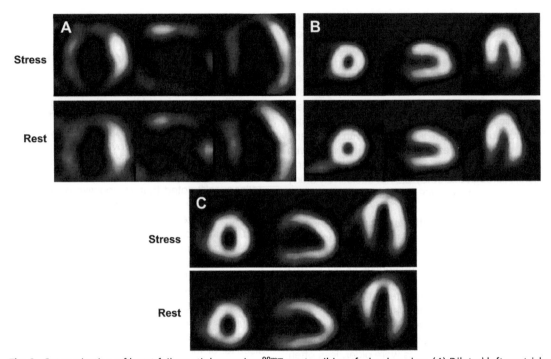

Fig. 8. Categorization of heart failure etiology using ^{99m}Tc-sestamibi perfusion imaging. (*A*) Dilated left ventricle with large, fixed perfusion defects in the septum, anterior wall, apex, and inferior wall suggestive of ischemic cardiomyopathy. (*B*) Normal stress-rest perfusion and left ventricular size indicative of heart failure related to diastolic mechanisms. (*C*) Dilated left ventricle and normal perfusion suggestive of nonischemic cardiomyopathy. These images demonstrate the value of myocardial perfusion imaging in excluding extensive coronary disease as the cause of heart failure. (*Adapted from* Soman P, Lahiri A, Mieres JH, et al. Etiology and pathophysiology of new-onset heart failure: evaluation by myocardial perfusion imaging. J Nucl Cardiol 2009;16(1):82–91; with permission.)

for patients with HF. Nuclear imaging modalities offer the only techniques with sufficient sensitivity to assess processes that take place at picomolar concentrations in the human heart,[70–72] thus providing potential valuable insights into the pathophysiology, severity, management response to treatment, and prognosis of HF patients.

Imaging of myocardial metabolism and viability

Iodine-123–labeled 15-(*p*-iodophenyl)-3-(*R,S*) methlypentadecanoic acid (^{123}I-BMIPP) is a branched-chain fatty acid with similar biodistribution, kinetics, and catabolism to long-chain fatty acids, but once inside the cells it is trapped intracellularly, due to enzymatic conversion. The presence of decreased myocardial ^{123}I-BMIPP uptake within normally perfused myocardium in SPECT imaging denotes ischemic jeopardized myocardium with decreased production of adenosine triphosphate derived from decreased β-oxidation of fatty acid.[73]

^{11}C-Acetate myocardial PET imaging allows assessment of the tricarboxylic acid cycle.[74] The early rapid clearance of acetate correlates closely with myocardial oxygen consumption, and the

relationship of myocardial ^{11}C-acetate kinetics to cardiac work offers a noninvasive parameter for cardiac efficiency that can be used to demonstrate the effect of pharmacologic and pacing interventions on cardiac energy.[75] PET imaging has also shown that treatment of HF patients with β-blockers results in a decrease in myocardial fatty acid metabolism without a significant chance in glucose use using the long-chain fatty acid ^{18}F-14-(*R,S*)-fluro-6-thia-heptadecanoic acid (^{18}F-FTHA) and ^{18}F-FDG.[76]

Imaging of myocardial dyssynchrony

Studies with ERNA have shown that phase analysis is useful for the evaluation of cardiac dyssynchrony. Based on the first Fourier harmonic fit of the blood pool time versus radioactivity curve, phase analysis allows the assessment of the time of ventricular contraction onset (expressed by the earliest ventricular phase angle), the mean time of the ventricular contraction onset (ie, the mean ventricular phase angle), and the synchrony of the ventricular contraction onset (ie, the standard deviation [SD] of the phase angle).[77] Furthermore, assessment of LV

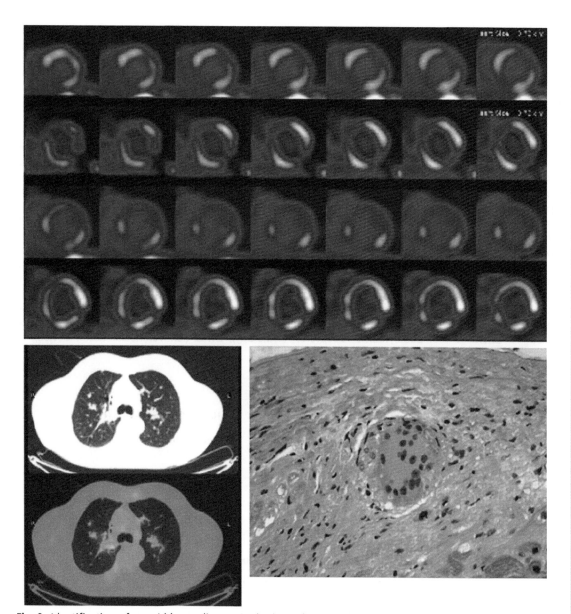

Fig. 9. Identification of sarcoid heart disease. Multiple perfusion defects on PET imaging do not correspond to coronary vascular territories. ^{18}F-FDG PET confirms the presence of increased metabolic activity in mediastinal lymph nodes. The diagnosis was confirmed on histologic examination. (*Reproduced from* Marwick TH, Schwaiger M. The future of cardiovascular imaging in the diagnosis and management of heart failure, part 2: clinical applications. Circ Cardiovasc Imaging 2008;1(2):162–70; with permission.)

dyssynchrony has also been approached with gated blood pool SPECT ventriculography[78] by the calculation of phase SD and phase delay between the left and right ventricles as the quantitative indices for interventricular and intraventricular dyssynchrony.

Recently, an automatic count-based method using gated SPECT MPI has been developed to assess the synchrony of LV mechanical contraction.[79] This method may have important clinical impact due to the widespread availability, automation, and reproducibility of gated SPECT MPI. Phase analysis of gated SPECT MPI has favorably been compared with other methods of measuring LV dyssynchrony.[80]

Imaging of myocardial interstitial dysregulation

Changes in the interstitium relate mainly to fibrosis. Myocardial fibrosis is dynamically determined by the equilibrium between fibroblast collagen synthesis and matrix metalloproteinase (MMP) collagen degradation. Both MMP2 (present in cardiomyocytes and fibroblasts) and MMP9 (present in inflammatory cells) are involved in ventricular remodeling.

Imaging of cardiac autonomic innervation

Cardiac autonomic function plays a crucial role in health and disease, with abnormalities both reflecting the severity of the disease and contributing specifically to clinical deterioration and poor prognosis. Radiotracer analogues of the sympathetic mediator norepinephrine have been investigated extensively, and are on the brink of potential widespread clinical use.[81]

The most widely studied SPECT tracer, ^{123}I-metaiodobenzylguanidine (^{123}I-mIBG), uses the same uptake, storage, and release mechanisms as norepinephrine in the sympathetic nerve endings. However, ^{123}I-mIBG is neither metabolized nor interacts with postsynaptic receptors, thus allowing in vivo scintigraphic visualization of the sympathetic postganglionic presynaptic fibers, as well as the assessment of both anatomic integrity and function of the nerve terminals.[70,71]

Cardiac ^{123}I-mIBG uptake is measured by defining the heart-to-mediastinum uptake ratio (HMR) at 15 minutes (early HMR) and 4 hours (late HMR) after tracer injection, and assessing washout kinetics (washout rate).[70,71] Planar and/or SPECT studies with ^{123}I-mIBG show reduced activity in the myocardium (low HMR and high washout rate) in patients with HF (**Fig. 10**).[82]

Increased global cardiac uptake appears to have a high NPV in terms of cardiac events, especially death and arrhythmias, and therefore and may have a role in guiding therapy, particularly by helping to better select patients unresponsive to conventional medical therapies who would benefit from device therapies such as an ICD (implantable cardioverter defibrillator), CRT (cardiac resynchronization therapy), LVAD (left ventricular assist device), or

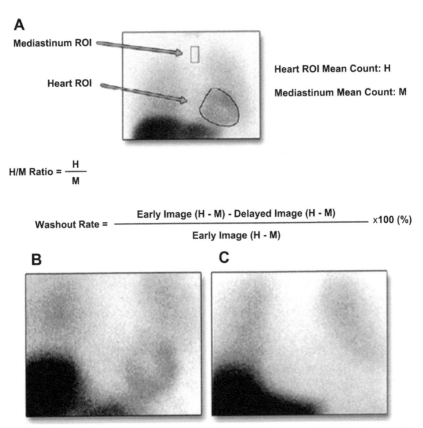

Fig. 10. Quantification of cardiac *meta*-iodobenzylguanidine (*m*IBG) activity. (A) Calculation of *m*IBG heart-to-mediastinum ratio (HMR) and washout rate on an anterior view of the thorax. Regions of interest (ROI) are drawn over the heart and mediastinum. (B) Normal cardiac *m*IBG activity in a patient with HMR of 1.80. (C) Severely decreased cardiac *m*IBG activity in a patient with HMR of 1.10. (*Reproduced from* Carrio I, Cowie MR, Yamazaki J, et al. Cardiac sympathetic imaging with mIBG in heart failure. JACC Cardiovasc Imaging 2010;3(1):92–100; with permission.)

cardiac transplantation. There are several studies showing [123]I-*m*IBG as an independent marker for cardiac events in patients with advanced symptomatic HF. Prospective data from the ADMIRE-HF study indicate that cardiac sympathetic imaging provides additional incremental prognostic value over measurements of LVEF and brain natriuretic peptide.[83]

At present, the data for [123]I-*m*IBG in stage B HF are limited. However, cardiac autonomic imaging with SPECT and PET tracers have shown potential in assessing patients following cardiac transplant, those with primary arrhythmic condition, those with CAD, and patients undergoing cardiotoxic chemotherapy. Cardiac sympathetic imaging with [123]I-*m*IBG provides a tool for better assessment of the diabetic heart.[84] The use of cardiac sympathetic imaging to risk-stratify this patient population is justified by the poor long-term prognosis of asymptomatic diabetic patients with cardiac autonomic neuropathy. Scholte and colleagues[85] examined the relationship between cardiac autonomic neuropathy, as determined using heart rate variability measurements and cardiac [123]I-*m*IBG imaging parameters, in diabetic patients without symptoms of coronary disease. A head-to-head comparison between [123]I-*m*IBG scintigraphy and heart rate variability measurements showed that [123]I-*m*IBG scintigraphy identifies significantly more patients with cardiac autonomic neuropathy than are identified by heart rate variability measurements. These findings provide further proof that [123]I-*m*IBG myocardial scintigraphy may have a role in the early detection of cardiac autonomic neuropathy. Radiotracer imaging of cardiac autonomic function allows visualization and quantitative measurements of underlying molecular aspects of cardiac disease, and should therefore provide a perspective that other cardiac tests cannot,[81] which is relevant especially in patients with ALVD.

SUMMARY

Radionuclide techniques such as gated SPECT MPI could be used as a one-stop shop for imaging patients with stage B HF/asymptomatic LV dysfunction. It could determine LV function, evaluate for the presence of obstructive CAD, determine the extent of viable myocardium, and evaluate dyssynchronous LV contraction. Radionuclide imaging can thus provide important noninvasive insights into the pathophysiology, prognosis, and management of patients with asymptomatic LV dysfunction as well as those with more advanced heat failure.

REFERENCES

1. Ghali JK, Cooper R, Ford E. Trends in hospitalization rates for heart failure in the United States, 1973-1986. Evidence for increasing population prevalence. Arch Intern Med 1990;150(4):769–73.
2. Gheorghiade M, Bonow RO. Chronic heart failure in the United States: a manifestation of coronary artery disease. Circulation 1998;97(3):282–9.
3. Goldberg LR, Jessup M. Stage B heart failure: management of asymptomatic left ventricular systolic dysfunction. Circulation 2006;113(24):2851–60.
4. Hunt SA, Abraham WT, Chin MH, et al. ACC/AHA 2005 Guideline Update for the Diagnosis and Management of Chronic Heart Failure in the Adult: a report of the American College of Cardiology/American Heart Association Task Force on Practice Guidelines (Writing Committee to Update the 2001 Guidelines for the Evaluation and Management of Heart Failure): developed in collaboration with the American College of Chest Physicians and the International Society for Heart and Lung Transplantation: endorsed by the Heart Rhythm Society. Circulation 2005;112(12):e154–235.
5. Frigerio M, Oliva F, Turazza FM, et al. Prevention and management of chronic heart failure in management of asymptomatic patients. Am J Cardiol 2003; 91(9A):4F–9F.
6. Wang TJ, Evans JC, Benjamin EJ, et al. Natural history of asymptomatic left ventricular systolic dysfunction in the community. Circulation 2003; 108(8):977–82.
7. Germano G, Kavanagh PB, Slomka PJ, et al. Quantitation in gated perfusion SPECT imaging: the Cedars-Sinai approach. J Nucl Cardiol 2007;14(4): 433–54.
8. Hyun IY, Kwan J, Park KS, et al. Reproducibility of TI-201 and Tc-99m sestamibi gated myocardial perfusion SPECT measurement of myocardial function. J Nucl Cardiol 2001;8(2):182–7.
9. Johnson LL, Verdesca SA, Aude WY, et al. Postischemic stunning can affect left ventricular ejection fraction and regional wall motion on post-stress gated sestamibi tomograms. J Am Coll Cardiol 1997;30(7):1641–8.
10. He J, Ogden LG, Bazzano LA, et al. Risk factors for congestive heart failure in US men and women: NHANES I epidemiologic follow-up study. Arch Intern Med 2001;161(7):996–1002.
11. Effect of enalapril on mortality and the development of heart failure in asymptomatic patients with reduced left ventricular ejection fractions. The SOLVD Investigators. N Engl J Med 1992;327(10): 685–91.
12. Poole-Wilson PA, Swedberg K, Cleland JG, et al. Comparison of carvedilol and metoprolol on clinical outcomes in patients with chronic heart failure in

the Carvedilol Or Metoprolol European Trial (COMET): randomised controlled trial. Lancet 2003;362(9377):7–13.

13. Klocke FJ, Baird MG, Lorell BH, et al. ACC/AHA/ASNC guidelines for the clinical use of cardiac radionuclide imaging–executive summary: a report of the American College of Cardiology/American Heart Association Task Force on Practice Guidelines (ACC/AHA/ASNC Committee to Revise the 1995 Guidelines for the Clinical Use of Cardiac Radionuclide Imaging). J Am Coll Cardiol 2003;42(7):1318–33.

14. Udelson JE, Shafer CD, Carrio I. Radionuclide imaging in heart failure: assessing etiology and outcomes and implications for management. J Nucl Cardiol 2002;9(Suppl 5):40S–52S.

15. Danias PG, Papaioannou GI, Ahlberg AW, et al. Usefulness of electrocardiographic-gated stress technetium-99m sestamibi single-photon emission computed tomography to differentiate ischemic from nonischemic cardiomyopathy. Am J Cardiol 2004;94(1):14–9.

16. Soman P, Lahiri A, Mieres JH, et al. Etiology and pathophysiology of new-onset heart failure: evaluation by myocardial perfusion imaging. J Nucl Cardiol 2009;16(1):82–91.

17. Wu YW, Yen RF, Chieng PU, et al. Tl-201 myocardial SPECT in differentiation of ischemic from nonischemic dilated cardiomyopathy in patients with left ventricular dysfunction. J Nucl Cardiol 2003;10(4):369–74.

18. Doi YL, Chikamori T, Tukata J, et al. Prognostic value of thallium-201 perfusion defects in idiopathic dilated cardiomyopathy. Am J Cardiol 1991;67(2):188–93.

19. Soman P, Dave DM, Udelson JE, et al. Vascular endothelial dysfunction is associated with reversible myocardial perfusion defects in the absence of obstructive coronary artery disease. J Nucl Cardiol 2006;13(6):756–60.

20. Heller GV, Links J, Bateman TM, et al. American Society of Nuclear Cardiology and Society of Nuclear Medicine joint position statement: attenuation correction of myocardial perfusion SPECT scintigraphy. J Nucl Cardiol 2004;11(2):229–30.

21. Naya M, Di Carli MF. Myocardial perfusion PET/CT to evaluate known and suspected coronary artery disease. Q J Nucl Med Mol Imaging 2010;54(2):145–56.

22. Berman DS, Shaw LJ, Min JK, et al. SPECT/PET myocardial perfusion imaging versus coronary CT angiography in patients with known or suspected CAD. Q J Nucl Med Mol Imaging 2010;54(2):177–200.

23. Gaemperli O, Kaufmann PA. Multimodality cardiac imaging. J Nucl Cardiol 2010;17(1):4–7.

24. Knuuti J, Kajander S, Maki M, et al. Quantification of myocardial blood flow will reform the detection of CAD. J Nucl Cardiol 2009;16(4):497–506.

25. Muhlbaier LH, Pryor DB, Rankin JS, et al. Observational comparison of event-free survival with medical and surgical therapy in patients with coronary artery disease. 20 years of follow-up. Circulation 1992;86(Suppl 5):II198–204.

26. Di Carli MF, Asgarzadie F, Schelbert HR, et al. Quantitative relation between myocardial viability and improvement in heart failure symptoms after revascularization in patients with ischemic cardiomyopathy. Circulation 1995;92(12):3436–44.

27. Marwick TH, Zuchowski C, Lauer MS, et al. Functional status and quality of life in patients with heart failure undergoing coronary bypass surgery after assessment of myocardial viability. J Am Coll Cardiol 1999;33(3):750–8.

28. Bax JJ, Poldermans D, Elhendy A, et al. Improvement of left ventricular ejection fraction, heart failure symptoms and prognosis after revascularization in patients with chronic coronary artery disease and viable myocardium detected by dobutamine stress echocardiography. J Am Coll Cardiol 1999;34(1):163–9.

29. Bax JJ, Wijns W, Cornel JH, et al. Accuracy of currently available techniques for prediction of functional recovery after revascularization in patients with left ventricular dysfunction due to chronic coronary artery disease: comparison of pooled data. J Am Coll Cardiol 1997;30(6):1451–60.

30. Kim RJ, Wu E, Rafael A, et al. The use of contrast-enhanced magnetic resonance imaging to identify reversible myocardial dysfunction. N Engl J Med 2000;343(20):1445–53.

31. Meluzin J, Cigarroa CG, Brickner ME, et al. Dobutamine echocardiography in predicting improvement in global left ventricular systolic function after coronary bypass or angioplasty in patients with healed myocardial infarcts. Am J Cardiol 1995;76(12):877–80.

32. Senior R, Kaul S, Raval U, et al. Impact of revascularization and myocardial viability determined by nitrate-enhanced Tc-99m sestamibi and Tl-201 imaging on mortality and functional outcome in ischemic cardiomyopathy. J Nucl Cardiol 2002;9(5):454–62.

33. Allman KC, Shaw LJ, Hachamovitch R, et al. Myocardial viability testing and impact of revascularization on prognosis in patients with coronary artery disease and left ventricular dysfunction: a meta-analysis. J Am Coll Cardiol 2002;39(7):1151–8.

34. Pagley PR, Beller GA, Watson DD, et al. Improved outcome after coronary bypass surgery in patients with ischemic cardiomyopathy and residual myocardial viability. Circulation 1997;96(3):793–800.

35. Senior R, Lahiri A, Kaul S. Effect of revascularization on left ventricular remodeling in patients with heart

failure from severe chronic ischemic left ventricular dysfunction. Am J Cardiol 2001;88(6):624–9.

36. Bonow RO. Identification of viable myocardium. Circulation 1996;94(11):2674–80.

37. Samady H, Elefteriades JA, Abbott BG, et al. Failure to improve left ventricular function after coronary revascularization for ischemic cardiomyopathy is not associated with worse outcome. Circulation 1999;100(12):1298–304.

38. Myers JH, Stirling MC, Choy M, et al. Direct measurement of inner and outer wall thickening dynamics with epicardial echocardiography. Circulation 1986;74(1):164–72.

39. Lieberman AN, Weiss JL, Jugdutt BI, et al. Two-dimensional echocardiography and infarct size: relationship of regional wall motion and thickening to the extent of myocardial infarction in the dog. Circulation 1981;63(4):739–46.

40. Kaul S. There may be more to myocardial viability than meets the eye. Circulation 1995;92(10): 2790–3.

41. Schinkel AF, Poldermans D, Elhendy A, et al. Assessment of myocardial viability in patients with heart failure. J Nucl Med 2007;48(7):1135–46.

42. Schinkel AF, Bax JJ, Delgado V, et al. Clinical relevance of hibernating myocardium in ischemic left ventricular dysfunction. Am J Med 2010;123(11): 978–86.

43. Pohost GM, Zir LM, Moore RH, et al. Differentiation of transiently ischemic from infarcted myocardium by serial imaging after a single dose of thallium-201. Circulation 1977;55(2):294–302.

44. Bonow RO, Dilsizian V. Thallium-201 and technetium-99m-sestamibi for assessing viable myocardium. J Nucl Med 1992;33(5):815–8.

45. Udelson JE, Coleman PS, Metherall J, et al. Predicting recovery of severe regional ventricular dysfunction. Comparison of resting scintigraphy with 201Tl and 99mTc-sestamibi. Circulation 1994;89(6): 2552–61.

46. Sciagra R, Bisi G, Santoro GM, et al. Comparison of baseline-nitrate technetium-99m sestamibi with rest-redistribution thallium-201 tomography in detecting viable hibernating myocardium and predicting post-revascularization recovery. J Am Coll Cardiol 1997; 30(2):384–91.

47. Auerbach MA, Schoder H, Hoh C, et al. Prevalence of myocardial viability as detected by positron emission tomography in patients with ischemic cardiomyopathy. Circulation 1999;99(22):2921–6.

48. Cleland JG, Pennell DJ, Ray SG, et al. Myocardial viability as a determinant of the ejection fraction response to carvedilol in patients with heart failure (CHRISTMAS trial): randomised controlled trial. Lancet 2003;362(9377):14–21.

49. Camici PG, Wijns W, Borgers M, et al. Pathophysiological mechanisms of chronic reversible left ventricular dysfunction due to coronary artery disease (hibernating myocardium). Circulation 1997;96(9):3205–14.

50. Wijns W, Vatner SF, Camici PG. Hibernating myocardium. N Engl J Med 1998;339(3):173–81.

51. Ragosta M, Beller GA, Watson DD, et al. Quantitative planar rest-redistribution ^{201}Tl imaging in detection of myocardial viability and prediction of improvement in left ventricular function after coronary bypass surgery in patients with severely depressed left ventricular function. Circulation 1993;87(5):1630–41.

52. Camici PG, Prasad SK, Rimoldi OE. Stunning, hibernation, and assessment of myocardial viability. Circulation 2008;117(1):103–14.

53. Slart RH, Bax JJ, de Boer J, et al. Comparison of ^{99m}Tc-sestamibi/[18]FDG DISA SPECT with PET for the detection of viability in patients with coronary artery disease and left ventricular dysfunction. Eur J Nucl Med Mol Imaging 2005;32(8):972–9.

54. Chareonthaitawee P, Christian TF, Hirose K, et al. Relation of initial infarct size to extent of left ventricular remodeling in the year after acute myocardial infarction. J Am Coll Cardiol 1995;25(3):567–73.

55. Christian TF, Behrenbeck T, Gersh BJ, et al. Relation of left ventricular volume and function over one year after acute myocardial infarction to infarct size determined by technetium-99m sestamibi. Am J Cardiol 1991;68(1):21–6.

56. Christian TF, Behrenbeck T, Pellikka PA, et al. Mismatch of left ventricular function and infarct size demonstrated by technetium-99m isonitrile imaging after reperfusion therapy for acute myocardial infarction: identification of myocardial stunning and hyperkinesia. J Am Coll Cardiol 1990;16(7): 1632–8.

57. Rahimtoola SH. A perspective on the three large multicenter randomized clinical trials of coronary bypass surgery for chronic stable angina. Circulation 1985;72(6 Pt 2):V123–35.

58. Elefteriades JA, Tolis G Jr, Levi E, et al. Coronary artery bypass grafting in severe left ventricular dysfunction: excellent survival with improved ejection fraction and functional state. J Am Coll Cardiol 1993;22(5):1411–7.

59. Rizzello V, Poldermans D, Biagini E, et al. Prognosis of patients with ischaemic cardiomyopathy after coronary revascularisation: relation to viability and improvement in left ventricular ejection fraction. Heart 2009;95(15):1273–7.

60. Eitzman D, al-Aouar Z, Kanter HL, et al. Clinical outcome of patients with advanced coronary artery disease after viability studies with positron emission tomography. J Am Coll Cardiol 1992;20(3):559–65.

61. Di Carli MF, Davidson M, Little R, et al. Value of metabolic imaging with positron emission tomography for evaluating prognosis in patients with coronary artery

disease and left ventricular dysfunction. Am J Cardiol 1994;73(8):527–33.

62. Stevenson WG, Stevenson LW, Middlekauff HR, et al. Improving survival for patients with advanced heart failure: a study of 737 consecutive patients. J Am Coll Cardiol 1995;26(6):1417–23.

63. Siebelink HM, Blanksma PK, Crijns HJ, et al. No difference in cardiac event-free survival between positron emission tomography-guided and single-photon emission computed tomography-guided patient management: a prospective, randomized comparison of patients with suspicion of jeopardized myocardium. J Am Coll Cardiol 2001;37(1):81–8.

64. Schinkel AF, Poldermans D, Rizzello V, et al. Why do patients with ischemic cardiomyopathy and a substantial amount of viable myocardium not always recover in function after revascularization? J Thorac Cardiovasc Surg 2004;127(2):385–90.

65. Soman P. Gated SPECT myocardial perfusion scintigraphy: a multi-faceted tool for the evaluation of heart failure. J Nucl Cardiol 2009;16(2):173–5.

66. Candell-Riera J, Romero-Farina G, Aguade-Bruix S, et al. Prognostic value of myocardial perfusion-gated SPECT in patients with ischemic cardiomyopathy. J Nucl Cardiol 2009;16(2):212–21.

67. Sharir T. Role of regional myocardial dysfunction by gated myocardial perfusion SPECT in the prognostic evaluation of patients with coronary artery disease. J Nucl Cardiol 2005;12(1):5–8.

68. Curtis JP, Sokol SI, Wang Y, et al. The association of left ventricular ejection fraction, mortality, and cause of death in stable outpatients with heart failure. J Am Coll Cardiol 2003;42(4):736–42.

69. Felker GM, Shaw LK, O'Connor CM. A standardized definition of ischemic cardiomyopathy for use in clinical research. J Am Coll Cardiol 2002;39(2):210–8.

70. Flotats A, Carrio I. Cardiac neurotransmission SPECT imaging. J Nucl Cardiol 2004;11(5):587–602.

71. Carrio I. Cardiac neurotransmission imaging. J Nucl Med 2001;42(7):1062–76.

72. Bengel FM, Schwaiger M. Assessment of cardiac sympathetic neuronal function using PET imaging. J Nucl Cardiol 2004;11(5):603–16.

73. Kawai Y, Tsukamoto E, Nozaki Y, et al. Significance of reduced uptake of iodinated fatty acid analogue for the evaluation of patients with acute chest pain. J Am Coll Cardiol 2001;38(7):1888–94.

74. Buxton DB, Schwaiger M, Nguyen A, et al. Radiolabeled acetate as a tracer of myocardial tricarboxylic acid cycle flux. Circ Res 1988;63(3):628–34.

75. Lindner O, Sorensen J, Vogt J, et al. Cardiac efficiency and oxygen consumption measured with ^{11}C-acetate PET after long-term cardiac resynchronization therapy. J Nucl Med 2006;47(3):378–83.

76. Wallhaus TR, Taylor M, DeGrado TR, et al. Myocardial free fatty acid and glucose use after carvedilol treatment in patients with congestive heart failure. Circulation 2001;103(20):2441–6.

77. Botvinick EH. Scintigraphic blood pool and phase image analysis: the optimal tool for the evaluation of resynchronization therapy. J Nucl Cardiol 2003;10(4):424–8.

78. Vilain D, Daou D, Casset-Senon D, et al. Optimal 3-dimensional method for right and left ventricular Fourier phase analysis in electrocardiography-gated blood-pool SPECT. J Nucl Cardiol 2001;8(3):371–8.

79. Chen J, Garcia EV, Folks RD, et al. Onset of left ventricular mechanical contraction as determined by phase analysis of ECG-gated myocardial perfusion SPECT imaging: development of a diagnostic tool for assessment of cardiac mechanical dyssynchrony. J Nucl Cardiol 2005;12(6):687–95.

80. Marsan NA, Henneman MM, Chen J, et al. Left ventricular dyssynchrony assessed by two three-dimensional imaging modalities: phase analysis of gated myocardial perfusion SPECT and tri-plane tissue Doppler imaging. Eur J Nucl Med Mol Imaging 2008;35(1):166–73.

81. Ji SY, Travin MI. Radionuclide imaging of cardiac autonomic innervation. J Nucl Cardiol 2010;17(4):655–66.

82. Carrio I, Cowie MR, Yamazaki J, et al. Cardiac sympathetic imaging with mIBG in heart failure. JACC Cardiovasc Imaging 2010;3(1):92–100.

83. Jacobson AF, Senior R, Cerqueira MD, et al. Myocardial iodine-123 meta-iodobenzylguanidine imaging and cardiac events in heart failure. Results of the prospective ADMIRE-HF (AdreView Myocardial Imaging for Risk Evaluation in Heart Failure) study. J Am Coll Cardiol 2010;55(20):2212–21.

84. Carrio I, Flotats A. Cardiac sympathetic imaging with mIBG: a tool for better assessment of the diabetic heart. Eur J Nucl Med Mol Imaging 2010;37(9):1696–7.

85. Scholte AJ, Schuijf JD, Delgado V, et al. Cardiac autonomic neuropathy in patients with diabetes and no symptoms of coronary artery disease: comparison of ^{123}I-metaiodobenzylguanidine myocardial scintigraphy and heart rate variability. Eur J Nucl Med Mol Imaging 2010;37(9):1698–705.

Biomarkers

Viorel G. Florea, MD, PhD, ScD[a,b,*],
Inder S. Anand, MD, FRCP, DPhil (Oxon)[a,b]

KEYWORDS

- Heart failure • Biomarkers • Brain natriuretic peptide
- Troponin

Biomarkers are biologic variables, the measurement of which provides information about a condition of interest. The term biomarker in heart failure is now applied to circulating serum and plasma analytes beyond the hematology and biochemistry included in routine clinical management. This term encompasses an expanding array of biochemical variables, the levels of which may reflect various aspects of the pathophysiology of heart failure.

Testing of clinical biomarkers in the setting of heart failure has 3 important goals[1]: (1) to identify possible underlying (and potentially reversible) causes of heart failure; (2) to confirm the presence or absence of the heart failure syndrome; and (3) to estimate the severity of heart failure and risk of disease progression. These objectives in no way detract from the other major benefit that may be expected from measuring biomarkers, that is, pathophysiologic insight. By reflecting the disease processes occurring at the whole body, organ, cellular, or intracellular levels, biomarkers may pinpoint potential novel therapeutic targets without being particularly powerful diagnostic or prognostic measures.

Putative biomarkers can be broadly classified into biomarkers of: (1) neurohormonal activation, (2) myocyte injury, (3) extracellular matrix remodeling, (4) inflammation, (5) renal dysfunction, (6) hematological abnormalities, (7) oxidative stress, and (8) those with less well-defined pathophysiologic associations (**Box 1**). Over the last decade, natriuretic peptides, particularly brain natriuretic peptide (BNP) and its aminoterminal cometabolite,

NT-proBNP, have been shown to be particularly useful in confirming or refuting the diagnosis of heart failure as well as stratifying long-term risk profiles. Several novel cardiac, metabolic, and inflammatory biomarkers have emerged in the heart failure literature (see **Box 1**), such as C-type natriuretic peptide,[2] midregional pro-A-type natriuretic peptide,[3,4] endothelin-1,[5] cardiac troponin and high-sensitivity troponin,[6,7] high-sensitivity C-reactive protein (hsCRP),[8–10] apelin,[11,12] myotrophin,[13] urotensin II,[14–16] adrenomedullin[17,18] and midregional proadrenomedullin,[3,19] cardiotrophin-1,[20,21] urocortin,[22] soluble ST2 receptor,[23] myeloperoxidase (MPO),[24] copeptin,[3,25] growth differentiation factor-15 (GDF-15),[26,27] lymphocyte G-protein coupled receptor kinases,[28] galectin-3,[29] and many others. Although their clinical role remains to be determined and validated, they characterize the various mechanisms of the development of left ventricular remodeling and dysfunction. Although a detailed appraisal of every proposed biomarker is beyond the scope of this review, we limit the discussion to the usefulness of biomarkers in patients with asymptomatic left ventricular dysfunction and stage B heart failure, with an emphasis on those with the greatest body of evidence.

BIOMARKERS OF NEUROHORMONAL ACTIVATION

It is now generally recognized that heart failure progresses through a process of structural

---

The authors have nothing to disclose.
[a] Department of Medicine, University of Minnesota Medical School, 420 Delaware Street Southeast, MMC 508, Minneapolis, MN 55455, USA
[b] Heart Failure Program, Cardiology 111-C, Minneapolis Veterans Affairs Health Care System, 1 Veterans Drive, Minneapolis, MN 55417, USA
* Corresponding author. Cardiology 111-C, Minneapolis Veterans Affairs Health Care System, 1 Veterans Drive, Minneapolis, MN 55417.
E-mail address: flore022@umn.edu

Box 1
Putative biomarkers in heart failure

Neurohormonal activation

B-type natriuretic peptide (BNP)

NT-proBNP

Atrial natriuretic peptide (ANP)

Norepinephrine

Endothelin

Adrenomedullin

Urocortin

Apelin

Plasma renin activity

Angiotensin II

Aldosterone

Arginine vasopressin

Myocyte injury

Cardiac troponin I (TnI)

Cardiac troponin T (TnT)

Heart-type fatty acid-binding protein

Myosin light chain-1

Extracellular matrix remodeling

Matrix metalloproteinases (MMPs)

Tissue inhibitors of metalloproteinases (TIMPs)

Inflammation

CRP

Tumor necrosis factor α (TNF-α)

Interleukins 1, 6, and 18 (IL-1, IL-6, IL-18)

Adhesion molecules

ST2

Oxidative stress

MPO

Urinary byopyrrins

Urinary and plasma isoprostanes

8-Epi-prostaglandin-F-α

Reduced glutathione/oxidized glutathione ratio

Plasma malondialdehyde

New biomarkers

Osteoprotegerin

Galectin-3

Chromogranin A

Adipokines

  Adiponectin

  Leptin

  Resistin

GDF-15

---

remodeling of the heart to which neurohormonal activation makes an important contribution.[30] Several lines of evidence support the role of neurohormones in the development of left ventricular dysfunction and heart failure. Norepinephrine[31] and angiotensin II[32] are directly toxic to cardiac myocytes. The degree of neurohormonal activation in heart failure is proportional to disease severity, increases with the progression of heart failure, and is related to prognosis.[33] Furthermore, changes in neurohormonal activation over time, occurring either spontaneously or in response to pharmacologic therapy, are also associated with proportional changes in subsequent mortality and morbidity.[34] The spectacular success in reducing heart failure morbidity and mortality by inhibiting the sympathetic and renin-angiotensin-aldosterone systems with β-blockers, angiotensin-converting enzyme inhibitors, and aldosterone receptor antagonists further underscored the importance of neurohormonal activation in the progression of both asymptomatic left ventricular dysfunction[35] and overt heart failure.[36–40]

NATRIURETIC PEPTIDES

The concept of the heart as an endocrine organ was advanced about 3 decades ago with the discovery that the heart synthesized and secreted ANP.[41,42] The production and release of ANP and BNP was later shown from models of experimental and human heart failure.[43,44] These hormones have emerged as cardiac biomarkers that can aid in the diagnosis, prognosis, and management of heart failure.[45,46]

Within the heart, the BNP gene produces a 134–amino acid preproBNP precursor peptide, which after removal of a 26–amino acid signal peptide, results in the 108–amino acid prohormone, proBNP. Subsequently, the enzyme corin cleaves proBNP into the biologically active mature 32–amino acid, BNP (BNP 1–32) and a linear 76–amino acid N-terminal peptide, NT-proBNP (**Fig. 1**).[47] All studies suggest that mature BNP 1–32 binds to the natriuretic peptide A receptor, activates the production of the second messenger cyclic guanosine monophosphate (GMP), and mediates the biologic actions of BNP. These actions include natriuresis, vasodilatation, enhancement of ventricular relaxation, inhibition of fibroblast activation, and suppression of the renin-angiotensin-aldosterone system.

Most of the early studies of natriuretic peptides have focused on the role of BNP or NT-proBNP testing among patients presenting with signs and symptoms of heart failure (stage C and D heart failure). As seen in **Box 2**,[46] natriuretic peptide

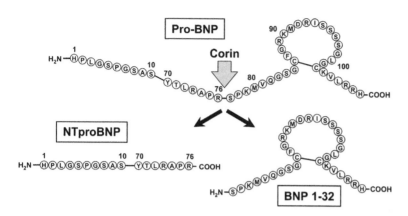

Fig. 1. Cleavage of proBNP into NT-proBNP and BNP. (*Adapted from* Boerrigter G, Costello-Boerrigter LC, Burnett JC. Natriuretic peptides in the diagnosis and management of chronic heart failure. Heart Fail Clin 2009;5:502; with permission.)

levels are currently used for diagnosis of acute decompensated heart failure, for confirmation of the heart failure diagnosis, and for risk stratification of patients with heart failure.[46] Repeat measurements of BNP or NT-proBNP levels have been used to guide treatment decisions in chronic heart failure.[48–52] BNPs have also been shown to have the potential to be useful surrogate end points in heart failure trials.[53,54]

The diagnostic and prognostic usefulness of plasma natriuretic peptide levels in the overt heart failure setting has prompted interest in evaluation of these biomarkers as screening tools for patients with asymptomatic left ventricular dysfunction (stage B heart failure). Luchner and colleagues[55] evaluated BNP as a marker of left ventricular dysfunction and hypertrophy in a population-based sample of 610 middle-aged individuals and showed that compared with individuals with normal left ventricular function and mass, individuals with left ventricular dysfunction or hypertrophy had increased BNP levels. Recent data from Olmsted County, Minnesota, showed that in stage A and B heart failure, plasma NT-proBNP values greater than age-specific/sex-specific 80th percentiles were associated with increased risk of death, heart failure, cerebrovascular accident, and myocardial infarction even after adjustment for clinical risk factors and structural cardiac abnormalities.[56] Higher NT-proBNP levels have also been associated with greater likelihood of detecting incident heart

---

Box 2
The role of natriuretic peptide levels in clinical practice

NP levels are quantitative plasma biomarkers of HF.

NP levels are accurate in the diagnosis of HF.

NP levels may help risk stratify patients in the ED with regard to the need for hospital admission or direct ED discharge.

NP levels help improve patient management and reduce total treatment costs in patients with acute dyspnea.

NP levels at the time of admission are powerful predictors of outcome in predicting death and rehospitalization in patients with HF.

NP levels at discharge aid in risk stratification of the patient with HF.

NP-guided therapy may improve morbidity or mortality in chronic HF.

The combination of NP levels together with symptoms, signs, and weight gain assists in the assessment of clinical decompensation in HF.

NP levels can accelerate accurate diagnosis of HF presenting in primary care.

NP levels may be helpful to screen for asymptomatic left ventricular dysfunction in high-risk patients.

Abbreviations: ED, emergency department; HF, heart failure; NP, natriuretic peptide.
   Adapted from Maisel A, Mueller C, Adams K Jr, et al. State of the art: using natriuretic peptide levels in clinical practice. Eur J Heart Fail 2008;10:824–39.

failure in a population with stable coronary artery disease.[57]

Recent investigations from the Framingham Heart Study reported that plasma natriuretic peptide levels predicted the risk of death and first cardiovascular event including heart failure, atrial fibrillation, and stroke or transient ischemic attack (**Fig. 2**). Excess risk was apparent at natriuretic peptide levels well below current thresholds used to diagnose heart failure.[58] However, the information obtained may be of limited clinical relevance by virtue of the lack of disease and diagnostic specificity and the lack of distinction between its use as a diagnostic or prognostic tool. In specific analyses, the accuracy of BNP or NT-proBNP in predicting future heart failure

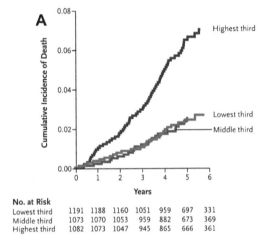

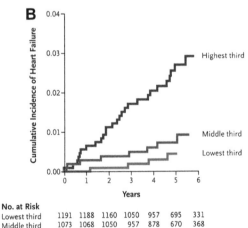

Fig. 2. Cumulative incidence of death (*A*) and heart failure (*B*), according to the plasma BNP level at base line. (*From* Wang T, Larson M, Levy D, et al. Plasma natriuretic peptide levels and the risk of cardiovascular events and death. N Engl J Med 2004;350:660; with permission.)

was generally suboptimal unless targeting high-risk groups.[59] The suboptimal diagnostic yield of BNP screening was also reported in a recent community-based study.[60] Using an empirically derived BNP cutoff of greater than 55 pg/mL to identify asymptomatic left ventricular systolic dysfunction (which had a prevalence of 1%), a positive test had a likelihood ratio of 3.8, whereas a negative test had a likelihood ratio of 0.1. In this population, using BNP as an initial screen would lead to referral for echocardiography in 24% of patients, 96% of whom would have no evidence of left ventricular dysfunction.[60] A recent pooled analysis of 3 large European epidemiologic studies used a different approach of defining an age-corrected and sex-corrected abnormal concentration of NT-proBNP, which was derived from normal individuals within a population of 3051 individuals.[61] When this analysis was applied to the entire population to detect heart failure and left ventricular systolic dysfunction, NT-proBNP emerged as an independent predictor of the presence of heart failure, with a sensitivity of 75% and a negative predictive value of 99%. This finding further reiterates the value of BNP/NT-proBNP testing as a rule-out, but questions the potential applicability of population screening using a test with only modest sensitivity. As a result, most guidelines do not support routine blood natriuretic peptide testing for screening large asymptomatic patient populations for left ventricular systolic dysfunction.[1]

Some investigators have attempted to increase the yield to detect asymptomatic left ventricular dysfunction by focusing on high-risk subgroups, a strategy that may be more cost-effective.[62] A high prevalence of increased plasma natriuretic peptide levels has been observed in a patient population at risk of developing heart failure (stage A heart failure), particularly among those with a history of long-term hypertension, diabetes mellitus,[63,64] coronary artery disease,[65,66] and in elderly individuals.[67–69] It is conceivable that blood natriuretic peptide testing may be useful for screening these high-risk populations who may otherwise be referred for further echocardiographic screening for asymptomatic left ventricular dysfunction, although the cutoff levels may differ in different patient populations. Others have combined several cardiac biomarkers to increase the specificity of screening using inflammatory markers such as MPO or hsCRP.[70] Until prospective studies are conducted to establish evidence for stratifying patients according to natriuretic peptide levels or to validate a multimarker approach with clinically available assays with cost-effectiveness justifications, broad clinical application of these approaches is still not warranted.[1]

BIOMARKERS OF MYOCYTE INJURY

Myocyte injury results from severe ischemia, but it is also a consequence of stresses on the myocardium such as inflammation, oxidative stress, and neurohormonal activation.

Cardiac Troponins

Troponins are proteins involved in the regulation of cardiac and skeletal muscle contraction. The cardiac troponin complex is made of TnI (inhibitory), troponin C (calcium binding), and TnT (tropomyosin binding) proteins. TnT is a 37-kD protein, tightly bound to the cardiac myofibrillar troponin-tropomyosin complex. TnI is a 24-kD protein, which decreases troponin C affinity for calcium, thus inhibiting troponin-tropomyosin interactions. Cardiac TnI, in particular, is not expressed by injured or regenerating skeletal muscle and is, therefore, exquisitely specific for myocardial injury.[71,72]

Measurement of circulating cardiac troponins plays a fundamental role in the diagnosis and management of the acute coronary syndromes.[73,74] In addition to their role in ischemic heart disease, accumulating data provide support for the importance of cardiac troponin measurement in heart failure.[7,75–78] In 1997, Missov and colleagues[79] were the first investigators to report increased levels of circulating cardiac TnI in patients with heart failure outside the context of clinically apparent ischemia. Multiple studies have subsequently examined the prevalence of transient or persistent increase of serum cardiac TnI or TnT levels in the setting of advanced heart failure[6,80] or in decompensated states.[81–83] Several clinical series have further shown a strong adverse prognostic effect of sustained increase of serial serum troponin levels, which may indicate ongoing myocardial damage.[84,85] **Fig. 3** shows the prognostic value of very low plasma concentrations of TnT in patients with stable chronic heart failure using both a standard and a high-sensitivity TnT assay.[7]

Multiple potential contributing mechanisms underlying cardiac troponin release in patients with heart failure have been proposed (**Fig. 4**), including subendocardial ischemia leading to myocyte necrosis, cardiomyocyte damage from inflammatory cytokines or oxidative stress, hibernating myocardium, or apoptosis.[75,86–89] In addition, cardiac troponin may be released from injured, but viable, myocardium as a result of increased permeability of the plasma membrane

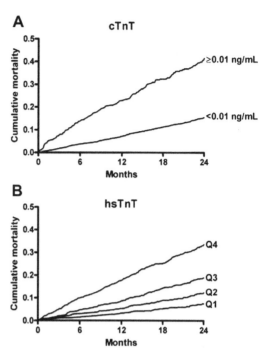

Fig. 3. Kaplan-Meier cumulative curves for mortality by baseline cardiac TnT (cTnT) (*A*) or by quartiles of high-sensitivity TnT (hsTnT) (*B*). For cTnT, log-rank = 224, *P*<.0001; for hsTnT, log-rank = 305, *P*<.0001. (*From* Latini R, Masson S, Anand IS, et al. Prognostic value of very low plasma concentrations of troponin T in patients with stable chronic heart failure. Circulation 2007;116:1245; with permission.)

and leakage of the cytosolic pool of cardiac troponin.[80,90]

Detectable circulating cardiac TnI is rare in the general population.[91] Recent data from a large observational study in Europe have shown an association between low levels of circulating cardiac troponin and the future development of heart failure in completely asymptomatic individuals (**Fig. 5**).[92] These data suggest that subclinical cardiomyocyte damage, as indicated by increased serum levels of cardiac TnI, may be an independent contributor to the development of heart failure in the community. Cardinale and colleagues[93,94] have shown that the increase in TnI soon after high-dose chemotherapy is a strong predictor of left ventricular dysfunction. These findings have important clinical implications in allowing the identification of patients at high risk of future cardiotoxicity in whom preventive measures are warranted. Circulating cardiac troponin may also provide insight into the transition from chronic compensated to acute decompensated heart failure. Biolo and colleagues[95] have recently reported that episodes of acute decompensated heart failure are associated with transient

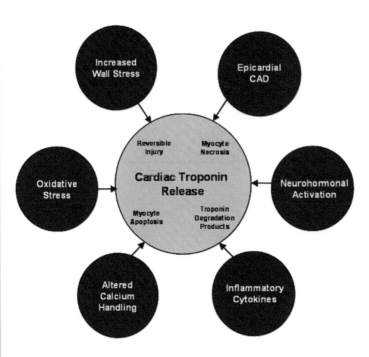

Fig. 4. Mechanisms of cardiac troponin release in heart failure. Multiple mechanisms may lead to myocyte necrosis, apoptosis, or reversible injury with increased myocyte membrane permeability, all resulting in cardiac troponin release. CAD, coronary artery disease. (*From* Kociol R, Pang P, Gheorghiade M, et al. Troponin elevation in heart failure. J Am Coll Cardiol 2010;56:1073; with permission.)

increases in markers of myocyte injury (plasma TnI) and extracellular matrix turnover (plasma MMPs, tissue inhibitors of MMPs, and procollagen N-terminal type I and procollagen type III N-terminal peptides) that may reflect an acceleration of pathologic myocardial remodeling during acute heart failure syndromes.[95]

The usefulness of routine assessment of serum troponin levels in patients with asymptomatic left ventricular systolic dysfunction or symptomatic heart failure, as well as the appropriate diagnostic and therapeutic approaches to increased serum troponin levels in nonacute coronary syndrome setting remains to be determined.

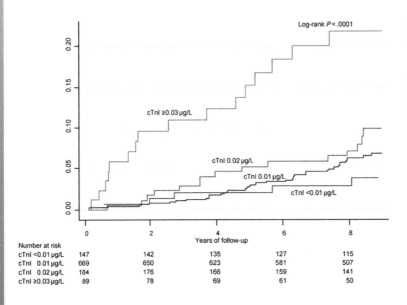

Fig. 5. Cumulative hazard of any heart failure by cardiac TnI groups. (*From* Sundstrom J, Ingelsson E, Berglund L, et al. Cardiac troponin-I and risk of heart failure: a community-based cohort study. Eur Heart J 2009;30:775; with permission.)

BIOMARKERS OF EXTRACELLULAR MATRIX REMODELING

The extracellular matrix of the heart is made up of several structural proteins, including fibrillar collagen, smaller amounts of elastin, and signaling peptides, laminin and fibronectin. The complex collagen three-dimensional weave, mainly consisting of type I collagen, interconnects individual myocytes through a collagen-integrin-cytoskeletal-myofibril arrangement. This network supports cardiac myocytes during contraction and relaxation and also provides a mechanism for translating individual myocyte shortening and force generation into ventricular contraction. It is also responsible for much of the passive diastolic stiffness of the ventricle.[96] In both human and animal studies, progressive left ventricular remodeling and dysfunction are associated with significant changes in the extracellular matrix.[97–100]

The structural hallmark of prolonged pressure-overload hypertrophy is significantly increased collagen accumulation between individual myocytes and myocyte fascicles (**Fig. 6**).[101,102] Thus, the highly organized architecture of the

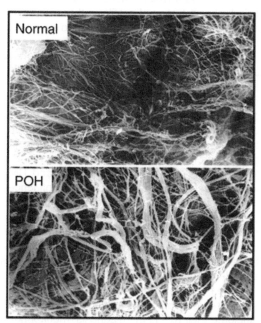

Fig. 6. Scanning electron micrographs taken from normal nonhuman primate left ventricular myocardium and after the induction of pressure overload hypertrophy (POH). These microscopic studies showed thickening of the collagen weave and overall increased relative content between myocytes with POH. (*From* Abrahams C, Janicki JS, Weber KT. Myocardial hypertrophy in Macaca fascicularis. Structural remodeling of the collagen matrix. Lab Invest 1987;56:676–83; with permission.)

extracellular matrix is replaced with a thickened, poorly organized extracellular matrix related to decreased capacity for extracellular matrix degradation and turnover. This reactive collagen deposition is characterized by both perivascular and interstitial fibrosis.[96,103,104] Enhanced synthesis and deposition of myocardial extracellular matrix in pressure-overload hypertrophy is directly associated with increased myocardial stiffness properties, which in turn causes poor filling characteristics during diastole.[102,105,106] Clinical evidence suggests that progressive extracellular matrix accumulation and diastolic dysfunction are important underlying pathophysiologic mechanisms for heart failure in patients with pressure-overload hypertrophy.[107,108]

In volume-overload hypertrophy caused by the persistently increased preload, a different pattern of extracellular matrix remodeling occurs. In large-animal models of volume-overload hypertrophy caused by chronic mitral regurgitation, the left ventricular remodeling process is accompanied by a distinctive loss of collagen fibrils surrounding individual myocytes.[109–111] These changes in extracellular matrix support are associated with changes in isolated left ventricular myocyte geometry, in which the cardiac cells increase in length. Representative scanning electron micrographs taken from a model of canine mitral regurgitation[109] can be seen in **Fig. 7** and show the profound differences in extracellular matrix structure and composition compared with normal myocardium and that of pressure-overload hypertrophy. Increased extracellular matrix proteolytic activity likely contributes to the reduced extracellular matrix content and support and thereby facilitates the overall left ventricular remodeling process.[112]

Although the mechanisms by which increased degradation of collagen promotes left ventricular dilatation and global left ventricular dysfunction are not clear, dissolution of the collagen weave may lead to increased elasticity and contribute to muscle fiber slippage and therefore an increase in chamber size.[105] Loss of collagen struts connecting individual myocytes could prevent transduction of individual myocyte contractions into myocardial force development, resulting in reduced myocardial systolic performance.

The extracellular matrix and, particularly, collagen are under dynamic control of 2 sets of proteins: those that favor degradation and those that tend to inhibit it. The dissolution or degradation of collagen is predominantly related to the activation of MMPs, a family of zinc-containing proteins that includes collagenases, gelatinases, stromelysins, and membrane-type MMPs.[112] Active

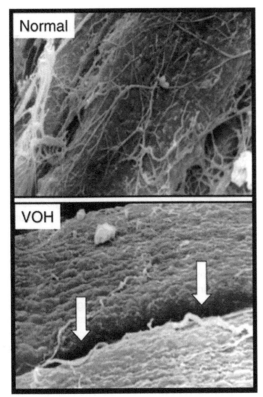

Fig. 7. Scanning electron micrographs taken from normal canine left ventricular myocardium after chronic mitral regurgitation that causes a volume overload hypertrophy (VOH). In this model of VOH, a loss of normal extracellular matrix architecture was shown between individual myocytes (*arrows*), and the collagen supporting network is poorly organized. (*From* Spinale FG. Myocardial matrix remodeling and the matrix metalloproteinases: influence on cardiac form and function. Physiol Rev 2007;87:1289; with permission.)

MMPs can undergo autodigestion and thereby lose proteolytic activity. However, the kinetics of this process are not fully understood and can be variable for different MMPs and conditions. A more critical control point for MMP activity is through the inhibition of the activated enzyme by the action of a group of specific MMP inhibitors termed TIMPs.[112] The TIMPs are low-molecular-weight proteins that can complex noncovalently with high efficiency to active MMPs, inhibiting their activity.[113,114]

Although the contributory mechanisms for the changes in plasma MMP and TIMPs levels remain speculative, these markers are regulated by several biologically active signal molecules such as angiotensin II, endothelin, reactive oxidant species and proinflammatory cytokines, all of which are strongly implicated in heart failure pathophysiology.[115]

Data from a Framingham Heart Substudy indicated that increased plasma MMP-9 levels were associated with left ventricular dilation.[116] Specifically, higher plasma levels of MMP-9 were associated with an approximately 2-fold higher risk of adverse left ventricular remodeling. Circulating levels of collagen degradation products have been associated with restrictive mitral filling patterns on echocardiography and poor prognosis in patients with dilated cardiomyopathy.[117] Other investigators have examined the role of polymorphisms in the genes for MMP-3 and MMP-9, which may influence prognosis in patients with established left ventricular systolic dysfunction.[118] The effects of MMPs are counterbalanced by TIMPs. In a community-based study of 1069 individuals, plasma levels of TIMP-1 were inversely associated with systolic function.[116] A recent study examined plasma levels of MMP-9 after acute myocardial infarction. Peak levels had independent predictive value for lower left ventricular ejection fraction during admission and for greater change in left ventricular dimensions between admission and follow-up.[119] In contrast, higher levels during follow-up were associated with relative preservation of left ventricular function and dimensions. This biphasic temporal profile, rather than absolute increase, in MMP-9 appeared to be related to the degree of left ventricular remodeling.

Changes in the plasma levels of TIMP-1 have been the focus of several large-scale cardiovascular outcome studies.[116,120] Increased TIMP-1 plasma levels have been associated with major cardiovascular risk factors and with the presence of left ventricular hypertrophy.[116] Furthermore, changes in plasma TIMP-1 levels have been associated with increased mortality.[120] However, it is likely that the changes in plasma MMP and TIMP levels observed in these studies are influenced by the underlying cause of the cardiovascular disease process, and therefore future studies are necessary. Although studies like these provide intriguing insights into the remodeling process, the application of MMP or TIMP monitoring as a viable biomarker of disease progression is questionable because of the limitations of routine analysis. Future proteomic strategies may further elucidate their role in the diagnosis, monitoring of disease progression, and prognostication of heart failure.

BIOMARKERS OF INFLAMMATION

The plasma levels of several inflammatory mediators have been found to be increased in patients with heart failure.[121] This finding led to the cytokine hypothesis, which holds that cytokines, like the neurohormones, may represent another class of biologically active molecules that are responsible for the development and progression of heart failure (**Fig. 8**).[122]

Interest in the presence of inflammatory mediators in patients with heart failure began in the 1950s, when a crude assay for CRP became available. Elster and colleagues[123] reported in 1956 that CRP was detectable in 30 of 40 patients with chronic heart failure and that heart failure was more severe in those with higher levels of CRP.[123] Since then, several cytokines have been implicated in the pathophysiology of heart failure. In 1990, Levine and colleagues[86] described increased levels of circulating TNF-α in patients with heart failure. In the Framingham Heart Study, inflammatory cytokines IL-6 and TNF-α as well as CRP were noted to identify asymptomatic older individuals in the community who were at high risk for the future development of heart failure.[124] Increased concentrations of both TNF and IL-6 have been associated with worsening symptoms, higher degree of exercise intolerance and neurohormonal activation and may also be predictive of outcome.[86,125–127] In a recent analysis of the Valsartan Heart Failure Trial (Val-HeFT), higher levels of CRP were associated with features of more severe heart failure, mortality, and morbidity.[9]

Circulating adhesion molecules are increased in heart failure. They play critical roles in the mediation of cell-cell interactions. For example, P-selectin mediates recruitment and migration of leukocytes beyond the endothelium leading to subsequent inflammatory infiltration.[128] Levels of intercellular adhesion molecule-1 and P-selectin are increased in heart failure when compared with healthy controls and seem to correlate with heart failure severity.[129]

Whether the increased concentrations of cytokines in heart failure are the result of, or a direct consequence of, heart failure has yet to be determined. Two approaches were recently used to antagonize the proinflammatory cytokine TNF-α in patients with heart failure: soluble TNF receptors and monoclonal antibodies; both approaches showed no benefit on clinical outcomes.[130] Routine measurement of cytokines presents several significant limitations. These proteins are released in other illnesses including infections. Intrapatient variations of IL-6 and TNF concentrations are broad. It remains to be proved whether routine measurement of cytokines would be clinically rewarding.

Although measurements of inflammatory mediators are not warranted for making specific therapeutic decisions in patients with acute or chronic heart failure, CRP levels were shown to augment the specificity of BNP in community screening for systolic heart failure.[70]

BIOMARKERS OF OXIDATIVE STRESS

Oxidative stress may be defined as a state of imbalance, whereby production of reactive oxygen species (ROS) exceeds endogenous antioxidant mechanisms (so-called nitroso-redox imbalance).

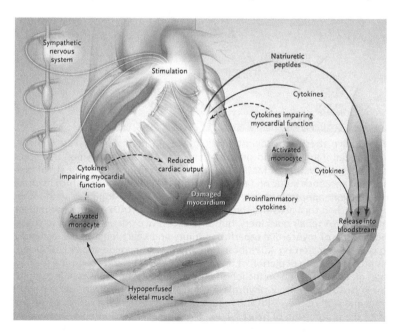

Fig. 8. The cytokine hypothesis of heart failure. According to the cytokine hypothesis of heart failure, proinflammatory cytokines (TNF-α, IL-1, IL-6, and IL-18) are produced by the damaged myocardium; this production is enhanced by stimulation of the sympathetic nervous system. Injured myocardium, as well as skeletal muscle that is hypoperfused because of reduced cardiac output, activates monocytes to produce the same cytokines, which act on and further impair myocardial function (*dashed lines*). Cytokines from these several sources are also released into the bloodstream. The stressed myocardium releases natriuretic peptides, denoted in red; their release improves the circulation. (*From* Braunwald E. Biomarkers in heart failure. N Engl J Med 2008; 358:2150; with permission.)

ROS include free radicals, such as superoxide anion ($O2^{\bullet-}$) and hydroxyl ($OH^{\bullet}$), as well as nonradical oxidants such as hydrogen peroxide (H_2O_2). These molecules are generated in most cell and tissue types, including the cardiovascular system.

The possible source of increased ROS in the failing myocardium include xanthine and reduced nicotinamide adenine dinucleotide phosphate oxidoreductases, cyclooxygenase, the mitochondrial electron transport chain, and activated neutrophils among many others.[131] The excessively produced nitric oxide (NO) derived from NO synthases has also been implicated in the pathogenesis of chronic heart failure (**Fig. 9**).[132] The combination of NO and superoxide yields peroxynitrite, a reactive oxidant, which has been shown to impair cardiac function via multiple mechanisms. Increased oxidative and nitrosative stress also activates the nuclear enzyme poly(ADP-ribose)

polymerase (PARP), which contributes to the pathogenesis of cardiac and endothelial dysfunction associated with myocardial infarction, chronic heart failure, diabetes, atherosclerosis, hypertension, aging, and various forms of shock. Recent studies have shown that pharmacologic inhibition of xanthine oxidase derived superoxide formation, neutralization of peroxynitrite, or inhibition of PARP provides significant benefit in various forms of cardiovascular injury.

Several indirect markers of oxidative stress have been shown to be altered in heart failure and to correlate with severity of myocardial dysfunction. The levels of plasma MPO[24] and isoprostane excretion correlate with the severity of heart failure and are independent predictors of heart failure mortality.[133] Urinary byopyrrins have been found to be increased in proportion to severity of left ventricular systolic dysfunction and New York Heart

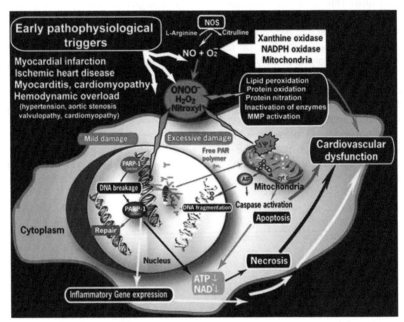

Fig. 9. Proposed role of oxidative/nitrosative stress and downstream pathway in heart failure. Peroxynitrite, formed from superoxide and NO, causes cell injury via lipid peroxidation, inactivation of enzymes and other proteins by oxidation and nitration, and also activation of MMPs. Peroxynitrite also triggers the release of pro-apoptotic factors such as cytochrome c and apoptosis inducing factor (AIF) from the mitochondria, which mediate caspase-dependent and caspase-independent apoptotic death pathways. Peroxynitrite together with other oxidants induces stand breaks in (DNA, which in turn activates the nuclear enzyme poly(ADP-ribose) polymerase (PARP). Mild damage of DNA activates the DNA repair machinery, but once excessive oxidative/nitrosative stress-induced damage occurs (like in various forms of myocardial reperfusion injury and heart failure), overactivated PARP initiates an energy-consuming cycle by transferring ADP-ribose units from nicotinamide adenine dinucleotide (NAD+) to nuclear proteins. This process leads to depletion of the intracellular NAD+ and adenosine triphosphate (ATP) pools, slowing the rate of glycolysis and mitochondrial respiration, eventually culminating to cardiovascular dysfunction or death. Poly(ADP-ribose) glycohydrolase (PARG) degrades poly(ADP-ribose) (PAR) polymers, generating free PAR polymer and ADP-ribose. PARP also regulates the expression of a variety of inflammatory mediators, which may facilitate the progression of heart failure. (*From* Ungvári Z, Gupte SA, Recchia FA, et al. Role of oxidative-nitrosative stress and downstream pathways in various forms of cardiomyopathy and heart failure. Curr Vasc Pharmacol 2005;3:225; with permission.)

Association functional class and correlate with BNP levels.[134] Similarly, other markers of oxidative stress have been shown to be increased in heart failure and show positive correlation with markers of neurohormonal activation and inflammation.[135–137] These novel markers can currently be measured using commercially available enzyme linked-immunosorbent or colorimetric assays.

Despite the experimental data supporting the role of ROS in development of the structural and functional changes in the myocardium during the progression of heart failure, the results of few controlled clinical trials with antioxidants such as vitamin C, a-tocopherol (vitamin E) and coenzyme Q10 are controversial. In some trials, antioxidant therapy was associated with improvement in myocardial function and symptoms, but in others, they exerted only mild or no effects on symptoms, ejection fraction, and exercise capacity.[138,139]

Some drugs that are being used in the treatment of heart failure, including angiotensin-converting enzyme inhibitors, statins, and the β-adrenergic antagonist carvedilol, may have important antioxidant properties. There is also evidence that the β-adrenergic antagonist metoprolol, which is not an antioxidant, can also decrease oxidative stress in patients with heart failure, raising the possibility that the effective treatment by decreasing cardiac overload could indirectly reduce oxidative stress.[138]

There is increasing evidence that xanthine oxidase, which catalyzes the production of 2 oxidants, hypoxanthine and xanthine, plays a pathologic role in heart failure.[140] There has been a longstanding recognition that increased serum uric acid is a surrogate marker for xanthine oxidase activity and a marker of chronic inflammation. It is also associated with impaired diastolic performance and poorer outcomes in both acute and chronic heart failure settings.[141–144] Increased levels of uric acid correlate with impaired hemodynamics[143,145] and independently predict an adverse prognosis in heart failure.[146] Although several studies suggested that inhibition of xanthine oxidase may improve endothelial reactivity,[147] myocardial function,[148] and ejection fraction[149] in patients with heart failure, in the OPT-CHF study (The Efficacy and Safety Study of Oxypurinol Added to Standard Therapy in Patients with New York Heart Association Class III–IV Congestive Heart Failure) oxypurinol did not produce clinical improvements in unselected patients with moderate to severe heart failure.[150]

Routine testing of the markers of oxidative stress is not used or warranted for making specific therapeutic decisions for patients with asymptomatic left ventricular dysfunction or acute or chronic heart failure.

NEW BIOMARKERS IN HEART FAILURE

New biomarkers continue to emerge from diverse aspects of the pathophysiology of heart failure.

Osteoprotegerin

Osteoprotegerin, a member of the TNF receptor superfamily, is a secreted glycoprotein with pleiotrophic functions, including the regulation of bone resorption.[151] Osteoprotegerin plays a regulatory role in inflammatory pathways,[152] acting as a decoy for the receptor activator of nuclear factor B ligand[151,153] and thus playing a role in promoting the activity of MMP, leading to degradation of extracellular matrix and increased apoptosis.[154] Increased serum levels of osteoprotegerin are present in humans who have ischemic and nonischemic heart failure[155] and correlate with the severity of heart failure, including higher New York Heart Association functional class, NT-proBNP level, and lower cardiac index.[154] Osteoprotegerin has been implicated in the development of subclinical left ventricular dysfunction (stage B heart failure).[156] In apparently healthy individuals from the community enrolled in the Dallas Heart Study, higher osteoprotegerin levels were associated with greater left ventricular mass and lower left ventricular ejection fraction.[156] Osteoprotegerin has also been shown to predict survival in patients with symptomatic heart failure after myocardial infarction.[155]

Galectin-3

Galectin-3, a protein produced by activated macrophages, is a member of a family of b-galactoside-binding lectins and promotes cardiac fibroblast proliferation and collagen synthesis.[29] Increased myocardial expression of galectin-3 is seen at an early stage in the progression of heart failure and may help to identify patients who have preclinical risk factors (stage A and B heart failure) who are more likely to develop overt heart failure.[29] In the Pro-BNP Investigation of Dyspnea in the Emergency Department study, higher levels of galectin-3 were observed in patients who had acute heart failure compared with those who had dyspnea from other causes.[157] In multivariate analysis adjusting for NT-proBNP, galectin-3 levels remained independently associated with 60-day mortality.[157] The combination of galectin-3 and NT-proBNP provided incremental prognostic information.[157]

Chromogranin A

Chromogranin A is a polypeptide present in the secretory granules throughout the neuroendocrine system.[158] Recent studies have shown increased myocardial expression of chromogranin A in patients with dilated and hypertrophic cardiomyopathy[159] as well as in patients with chronic heart failure from ischemic and nonischemic cardiomyopathy compared with healthy individuals.[159,160] Wohlschlaeger and colleagues[161] have recently reported decreased myocardial chromogranin A expression during reverse cardiac remodeling after ventricular unloading with a ventricular assist device. However, because of its low expression, the negative regulation of chromogranin A was not reflected by plasma levels and thus chromogranin A did not seem to be an appropriate biomarker of reverse cardiac remodeling after unloading.[161]

Adipokines

The metabolic abnormalities in chronic heart failure are accompanied by alterations in several biomarkers produced by adipose tissue (called adipokines), including adiponectin, leptin, and resistin. These adipokines exert local autocrine/paracrine effects on the myocardium in addition to systemic endocrine effects.[152] All of these adipokines are linked to cardiovascular diseases through their roles in regulation of energy balance, insulin sensitivity, angiogenesis, blood pressure, and lipid metabolism.[152]

GDF-15

GDF-15 is a distant member of the transforming growth factor β cytokine superfamily.[162] Accumulating evidence indicates that circulating levels of GDF-15 are associated with prognosis in patients with coronary artery disease[27] and chronic heart failure.[26,163]

We are now moving rapidly into the proteomic era, which provides a greatly expanded approach to the study of proteins, their variations, and their concentrations. The evaluation of proteins using mass spectrometric analysis coupled with high-pressure liquid chromatography is likely to yield new classes of biomarkers of asymptomatic left ventricular dysfunction and heart failure.[164]

Despite the intriguing early information from these newer markers, none is ready for clinical use. The biomarker field is becoming ever more crowded with candidate markers, and the pathway from early development to clinical application of biomarkers is appropriately steep. Whether measurement of these biomarkers early in the natural history of heart failure helps identify patients with stage B heart failure remains to be established. Considerable additional study is needed to determine how these biomarkers fit into diagnostic and treatment algorithms for patients with various stages of heart failure.

SUMMARY

Biomarkers reflect diverse aspects of the pathophysiology of asymptomatic left ventricular dysfunction and heart failure, including neurohormonal activation, myocyte stress and injury, inflammation, oxidative stress, and cellular and extracellular matrix remodeling.[75] To be clinically useful, a particular biomarker must provide diagnostic or prognostic information that is not readily available from careful clinical assessment, and aid in clinical decision making.[165] At present, only the natriuretic peptides seem to meet these clinical purposes and have recently made their way into heart failure practice guidelines.[1] The many other biomarkers receiving attention in asymptomatic left ventricular dysfunction and heart failure are of scientific interest, because they provide insight into the complex pathophysiology of the disease, suggesting new directions for fundamental research or the development of new therapies. Further advances in our understanding of currently available and future cardiac biomarkers will facilitate improved characterization of heart failure disease states and promote individualized therapy in heart failure and beyond.

REFERENCES

1. Tang WH, Francis GS, Morrow DA, et al. National Academy of Clinical Biochemistry Laboratory Medicine practice guidelines: clinical utilization of cardiac biomarker testing in heart failure. Circulation 2007;116(5):e99–109.
2. Kalra PR, Clague JR, Bolger AP, et al. Myocardial production of C-type natriuretic peptide in chronic heart failure. Circulation 2003;107(4):571–3.
3. Gegenhuber A, Struck J, Dieplinger B, et al. Comparative evaluation of B-type natriuretic peptide, mid-regional pro-A-type natriuretic peptide, mid-regional pro-adrenomedullin, and Copeptin to predict 1-year mortality in patients with acute destabilized heart failure. J Card Fail 2007;13(1):42–9.
4. Liang F, O'Rear J, Schellenberger U, et al. Evidence for functional heterogeneity of circulating B-type natriuretic peptide. J Am Coll Cardiol 2007; 49(10):1071–8.
5. Kinugawa T, Kato M, Ogino K, et al. Plasma endothelin-1 levels and clinical correlates in

patients with chronic heart failure. J Card Fail 2003; 9(4):318–24.

6. Horwich TB, Patel J, MacLellan WR, et al. Cardiac troponin I is associated with impaired hemodynamics, progressive left ventricular dysfunction, and increased mortality rates in advanced heart failure. Circulation 2003;108(7):833–8.

7. Latini R, Masson S, Anand IS, et al. Prognostic value of very low plasma concentrations of troponin T in patients with stable chronic heart failure. Circulation 2007;116(11):1242–9.

8. Alonso-Martinez JL, Llorente-Diez B, Echegaray-Agara M, et al. C-reactive protein as a predictor of improvement and readmission in heart failure. Eur J Heart Fail 2002;4(3):331–6.

9. Anand IS, Latini R, Florea VG, et al. C-reactive protein in heart failure: prognostic value and the effect of valsartan. Circulation 2005;112(10): 1428–34.

10. Berton G, Cordiano R, Palmieri R, et al. C-reactive protein in acute myocardial infarction: association with heart failure. Am Heart J 2003;145(6): 1094–101.

11. Chen MM, Ashley EA, Deng DX, et al. Novel role for the potent endogenous inotrope apelin in human cardiac dysfunction. Circulation 2003;108(12): 1432–9.

12. Foldes G, Horkay F, Szokodi I, et al. Circulating and cardiac levels of apelin, the novel ligand of the orphan receptor APJ, in patients with heart failure. Biochem Biophys Res Commun 2003; 308(3):480–5.

13. O'Brien RJ, Loke I, Davies JE, et al. Myotrophin in human heart failure. J Am Coll Cardiol 2003; 42(4):719–25.

14. Douglas SA, Tayara L, Ohlstein EH, et al. Congestive heart failure and expression of myocardial urotensin II. Lancet 2002;359(9322):1990–7.

15. Ng LL, Loke I, O'Brien RJ, et al. Plasma urotensin in human systolic heart failure. Circulation 2002; 106(23):2877–80.

16. Richards AM, Nicholls MG, Lainchbury JG, et al. Plasma urotensin II in heart failure. Lancet 2002; 360(9332):545–6.

17. Richards AM, Doughty R, Nicholls MG, et al. Plasma N-terminal pro-brain natriuretic peptide and adrenomedullin: prognostic utility and prediction of benefit from carvedilol in chronic ischemic left ventricular dysfunction. Australia-New Zealand Heart Failure Group. J Am Coll Cardiol 2001; 37(7):1781–7.

18. Richards AM, Nicholls MG, Yandle TG, et al. Plasma N-terminal pro-brain natriuretic peptide and adrenomedullin: new neurohormonal predictors of left ventricular function and prognosis after myocardial infarction. Circulation 1998;97(19): 1921–9.

19. Maisel A, Mueller C, Nowak R, et al. Mid-region pro-hormone markers for diagnosis and prognosis in acute dyspnea: results from the BACH (Biomarkers in Acute Heart Failure) trial. J Am Coll Cardiol 2010;55(19):2062–76.

20. Ng LL, O'Brien RJ, Demme B, et al. Non-competitive immunochemiluminometric assay for cardiotrophin-1 detects elevated plasma levels in human heart failure. Clin Sci (Lond) 2002;102(4):411–6.

21. Talwar S, Squire IB, Downie PF, et al. Elevated circulating cardiotrophin-1 in heart failure: relationship with parameters of left ventricular systolic dysfunction. Clin Sci (Lond) 2000;99(1):83–8.

22. Ng LL, Loke IW, O'Brien RJ, et al. Plasma urocortin in human systolic heart failure. Clin Sci (Lond) 2004;106(4):383–8.

23. Weinberg EO, Shimpo M, Hurwitz S, et al. Identification of serum soluble ST2 receptor as a novel heart failure biomarker. Circulation 2003;107(5): 721–6.

24. Tang WH, Brennan ML, Philip K, et al. Plasma myeloperoxidase levels in patients with chronic heart failure. Am J Cardiol 2006;98(6):796–9.

25. Stoiser B, Mortl D, Hulsmann M, et al. Copeptin, a fragment of the vasopressin precursor, as a novel predictor of outcome in heart failure. Eur J Clin Invest 2006;36(11):771–8.

26. Anand IS, Kempf T, Rector TS, et al. Serial measurement of growth-differentiation factor-15 in heart failure: relation to disease severity and prognosis in the Valsartan Heart Failure Trial. Circulation 2010;122(14):1387–95.

27. Kempf T, Sinning JM, Quint A, et al. Growth-differentiation factor-15 for risk stratification in patients with stable and unstable coronary heart disease: results from the AtheroGene study. Circ Cardiovasc Genet 2009;2(3):286–92.

28. Iaccarino G, Barbato E, Cipolletta E, et al. Elevated myocardial and lymphocyte GRK2 expression and activity in human heart failure. Eur Heart J 2005; 26(17):1752–8.

29. Sharma UC, Pokharel S, van Brakel TJ, et al. Galectin-3 marks activated macrophages in failure-prone hypertrophied hearts and contributes to cardiac dysfunction. Circulation 2004;110(19): 3121–8.

30. Anand IS, Florea VG. Alterations in ventricular structure: role of left ventricular remodeling. In: Mann DL, editor. Heart failure. A companion to Braunwald's heart disease. Philadelphia (PA): Saunders; 2004. p. 229–45.

31. Mann DL, Kent RL, Parsons B, et al. Adrenergic effects on the biology of the adult mammalian cardiocyte. Circulation 1992;85(2):790–804.

32. Tan LB, Jalil JE, Pick R, et al. Cardiac myocyte necrosis induced by angiotensin II. Circ Res 1991;69(5):1185–95.

33. Anand IS, Chandrashekhar Y. Neurohormonal responses in congestive heart failure: effect of ACE inhibitors in randomized controlled clinical trials. In: Dhalla NS, Singhal PK, Beamish RE, editors. Heart hypertrophy and failure. Boston: Kluwer Academic Publishers; 1996. p. 487–501.

34. Anand IS, Fisher LD, Chiang YT, et al. Changes in brain natriuretic peptide and norepinephrine over time and mortality and morbidity in the Valsartan Heart Failure Trial (Val-HeFT). Circulation 2003; 107(9):1278–83.

35. Effect of enalapril on mortality and the development of heart failure in asymptomatic patients with reduced left ventricular ejection fractions. The SOLVD Investigators. N Engl J Med 1992; 327(10):685–91.

36. Effects of enalapril on mortality in severe congestive heart failure. Results of the Cooperative North Scandinavian Enalapril Survival Study (CONSENSUS). The CONSENSUS Trial Study Group. N Engl J Med 1987;316(23):1429–35.

37. Effect of enalapril on survival in patients with reduced left ventricular ejection fractions and congestive heart failure. The SOLVD Investigators. N Engl J Med 1991;325(5):293–302.

38. Effect of metoprolol CR/XL in chronic heart failure: metoprolol CR/XL Randomised Intervention Trial in Congestive Heart Failure (MERIT-HF). Lancet 1999;353(9169):2001–7.

39. Packer M, Coats AJ, Fowler MB, et al. Effect of carvedilol on survival in severe chronic heart failure. N Engl J Med 2001;344(22):1651–8.

40. Pitt B, Zannad F, Remme WJ, et al. The effect of spironolactone on morbidity and mortality in patients with severe heart failure. Randomized Aldactone Evaluation Study Investigators. N Engl J Med 1999;341(10):709–17.

41. de Bold AJ, Borenstein HB, Veress AT, et al. A rapid and potent natriuretic response to intravenous injection of atrial myocardial extract in rats. Life Sci 1981;28(1):89–94.

42. Kangawa K, Matsuo H. Purification and complete amino acid sequence of alpha-human atrial natriuretic polypeptide (alpha-hANP). Biochem Biophys Res Commun 1984;118(1):131–9.

43. Burnett JC Jr, Kao PC, Hu DC, et al. Atrial natriuretic peptide elevation in congestive heart failure in the human. Science 1986;231(4742):1145–7.

44. Mukoyama M, Nakao K, Hosoda K, et al. Brain natriuretic peptide as a novel cardiac hormone in humans. Evidence for an exquisite dual natriuretic peptide system, atrial natriuretic peptide and brain natriuretic peptide. J Clin Invest 1991;87(4): 1402–12.

45. Maeda K, Tsutamoto T, Wada A, et al. Plasma brain natriuretic peptide as a biochemical marker of high left ventricular end-diastolic pressure in patients with symptomatic left ventricular dysfunction. Am Heart J 1998;135(5 Pt 1):825–32.

46. Maisel A, Mueller C, Adams K Jr, et al. State of the art: using natriuretic peptide levels in clinical practice. Eur J Heart Fail 2008;10(9):824–39.

47. Boerrigter G, Costello-Boerrigter LC, Burnett JC Jr. Natriuretic peptides in the diagnosis and management of chronic heart failure. Heart Fail Clin 2009; 5(4):501–14.

48. Coletta AP, Cullington D, Clark AL, et al. Clinical trials update from European Society of Cardiology meeting 2008: TIME-CHF, BACH, BEAUTIFUL, GISSI-HF, and HOME-HF. Eur J Heart Fail 2008; 10(12):1264–7.

49. Felker GM, Hasselblad V, Hernandez AF, et al. Biomarker-guided therapy in chronic heart failure: a meta-analysis of randomized controlled trials. Am Heart J 2009;158(3):422–30.

50. Jourdain P, Jondeau G, Funck F, et al. Plasma brain natriuretic peptide-guided therapy to improve outcome in heart failure: the STARS-BNP Multicenter Study. J Am Coll Cardiol 2007;49(16): 1733–9.

51. Lainchbury JG, Troughton RW, Strangman KM, et al. N-terminal pro-B-type natriuretic peptide-guided treatment for chronic heart failure: results from the BATTLESCARRED (NT-proBNP-Assisted Treatment To Lessen Serial Cardiac Readmissions and Death) trial. J Am Coll Cardiol 2009; 55(1):53–60.

52. Troughton RW, Frampton CM, Yandle TG, et al. Treatment of heart failure guided by plasma aminoterminal brain natriuretic peptide (N-BNP) concentrations. Lancet 2000;355(9210):1126–30.

53. Anand IS, Florea VG, Fisher L. Surrogate end points in heart failure. J Am Coll Cardiol 2002; 39(9):1414–21.

54. McDonagh T. Can BNP or NT-prp-BNP be considered surrogate end points for heart failure? Dialog Cardiovasc Med 2010;15(2):105–13.

55. Luchner A, Burnett JC Jr, Jougasaki M, et al. Evaluation of brain natriuretic peptide as marker of left ventricular dysfunction and hypertrophy in the population. J Hypertens 2000;18(8): 1121–8.

56. McKie PM, Cataliotti A, Lahr BD, et al. The prognostic value of N-terminal pro-B-type natriuretic peptide for death and cardiovascular events in healthy normal and stage A/B heart failure subjects. J Am Coll Cardiol 2010;55(19):2140–7.

57. Bibbins-Domingo K, Gupta R, Na B, et al. N-terminal fragment of the prohormone brain-type natriuretic peptide (NT-proBNP), cardiovascular events, and mortality in patients with stable coronary heart disease. JAMA 2007;297(2):169–76.

58. Wang TJ, Larson MG, Levy D, et al. Plasma natriuretic peptide levels and the risk of

cardiovascular events and death. N Engl J Med 2004;350(7):655–63.

59. Vasan RS, Benjamin EJ, Larson MG, et al. Plasma natriuretic peptides for community screening for left ventricular hypertrophy and systolic dysfunction: the Framingham heart study. JAMA 2002; 288(10):1252–9.

60. Costello-Boerrigter LC, Boerrigter G, Redfield MM, et al. Amino-terminal pro-B-type natriuretic peptide and B-type natriuretic peptide in the general community: determinants and detection of left ventricular dysfunction. J Am Coll Cardiol 2006; 47(2):345–53.

61. McDonagh TA, Holmer S, Raymond I, et al. NT-proBNP and the diagnosis of heart failure: a pooled analysis of three European epidemiological studies. Eur J Heart Fail 2004;6(3):269–73.

62. Nielsen OW, McDonagh TA, Robb SD, et al. Retrospective analysis of the cost-effectiveness of using plasma brain natriuretic peptide in screening for left ventricular systolic dysfunction in the general population. J Am Coll Cardiol 2003;41(1):113–20.

63. Epshteyn V, Morrison K, Krishnaswamy P, et al. Utility of B-type natriuretic peptide (BNP) as a screen for left ventricular dysfunction in patients with diabetes. Diabetes Care 2003;26(7):2081–7.

64. Silver MA, Pisano C. High incidence of elevated B-type natriuretic peptide levels and risk factors for heart failure in an unselected at-risk population (stage A): implications for heart failure screening programs. Congest Heart Fail 2003;9(3):127–32.

65. Richards M, Nicholls MG, Espiner EA, et al. Comparison of B-type natriuretic peptides for assessment of cardiac function and prognosis in stable ischemic heart disease. J Am Coll Cardiol 2006;47(1):52–60.

66. Tang WH, Steinhubl SR, Van Lente F, et al. Risk stratification for patients undergoing nonurgent percutaneous coronary intervention using N-terminal pro-B-type natriuretic peptide: a Clopidogrel for the Reduction of Events During Observation (CREDO) substudy. Am Heart J 2007;153(1):36–41.

67. Alehagen U, Lindstedt G, Eriksson H, et al. Utility of the amino-terminal fragment of pro-brain natriuretic peptide in plasma for the evaluation of cardiac dysfunction in elderly patients in primary health care. Clin Chem 2003;49(8):1337–46.

68. Groenning BA, Raymond I, Hildebrandt PR, et al. Diagnostic and prognostic evaluation of left ventricular systolic heart failure by plasma N-terminal pro-brain natriuretic peptide concentrations in a large sample of the general population. Heart 2004;90(3):297–303.

69. Hutcheon SD, Gillespie ND, Struthers AD, et al. B-type natriuretic peptide in the diagnosis of cardiac disease in elderly day hospital patients. Age Ageing 2002;31(4):295–301.

70. Ng LL, Pathik B, Loke IW, et al. Myeloperoxidase and C-reactive protein augment the specificity of B-type natriuretic peptide in community screening for systolic heart failure. Am Heart J 2006;152(1): 94–101.

71. Adams JE 3rd, Bodor GS, Davila-Roman VG, et al. Cardiac troponin I. A marker with high specificity for cardiac injury. Circulation 1993;88(1):101–6.

72. Bodor GS, Porterfield D, Voss EM, et al. Cardiac troponin-I is not expressed in fetal and healthy or diseased adult human skeletal muscle tissue. Clin Chem 1995;41(12 Pt 1):1710–5.

73. Kushner FG, Hand M, Smith SC Jr, et al. 2009 focused updates: ACC/AHA guidelines for the management of patients with ST-elevation myocardial infarction (updating the 2004 guideline and 2007 focused update) and ACC/AHA/SCAI guidelines on percutaneous coronary intervention (updating the 2005 guideline and 2007 focused update) a report of the American College of Cardiology Foundation/American Heart Association Task Force on Practice Guidelines. J Am Coll Cardiol 2009;54(23):2205–41.

74. Thygesen K, Alpert JS, White HD, et al. Universal definition of myocardial infarction. Circulation 2007;116(22):2634–53.

75. Braunwald E. Biomarkers in heart failure. N Engl J Med 2008;358(20):2148–59.

76. Kociol RD, Pang PS, Gheorghiade M, et al. Troponin elevation in heart failure prevalence, mechanisms, and clinical implications. J Am Coll Cardiol 2010;56(14):1071–8.

77. Latini R, Masson S, Anand IS, et al. High sensitivity troponin T is a strong predictor of outcomes in patients with chronic heart failure–a study from the Val-HeFT trial. Circulation 2005;112(Suppl 17):II-507.

78. Masson S, Latini R, Anand IS. An update on cardiac troponins as circulating biomarkers in heart failure. Curr Heart Fail Rep 2010;7(1):15–21.

79. Missov E, Calzolari C, Pau B. Circulating cardiac troponin I in severe congestive heart failure. Circulation 1997;96(9):2953–8.

80. Perna ER, Macin SM, Canella JP, et al. Ongoing myocardial injury in stable severe heart failure: value of cardiac troponin T monitoring for high-risk patient identification. Circulation 2004; 110(16):2376–82.

81. Macin SM, Perna ER, Cimbaro Canella JP, et al. Increased levels of cardiac troponin-T in outpatients with heart failure and preserved systolic function are related to adverse clinical findings and outcome. Coron Artery Dis 2006;17(8):685–91.

82. Perna ER, Macin SM, Cimbaro Canella JP, et al. Minor myocardial damage detected by troponin T is a powerful predictor of long-term prognosis in

patients with acute decompensated heart failure. Int J Cardiol 2005;99(2):253–61.

83. You JJ, Austin PC, Alter DA, et al. Relation between cardiac troponin I and mortality in acute decompensated heart failure. Am Heart J 2007;153(4): 462–70.

84. Stanton EB, Hansen MS, Sole MJ, et al. Cardiac troponin I, a possible predictor of survival in patients with stable congestive heart failure. Can J Cardiol 2005;21(1):39–43.

85. Taniguchi R, Sato Y, Nishio Y, et al. Measurements of baseline and follow-up concentrations of cardiac troponin-T and brain natriuretic peptide in patients with heart failure from various etiologies. Heart Vessels 2006;21(6):344–9.

86. Levine B, Kalman J, Mayer L, et al. Elevated circulating levels of tumor necrosis factor in severe chronic heart failure. N Engl J Med 1990;323(4): 236–41.

87. Logeart D, Beyne P, Cusson C, et al. Evidence of cardiac myolysis in severe nonischemic heart failure and the potential role of increased wall strain. Am Heart J 2001;141(2):247–53.

88. Narula J, Haider N, Virmani R, et al. Apoptosis in myocytes in end-stage heart failure. N Engl J Med 1996;335(16):1182–9.

89. Olivetti G, Abbi R, Quaini F, et al. Apoptosis in the failing human heart. N Engl J Med 1997;336(16): 1131–41.

90. Sato Y, Kita T, Takatsu Y, et al. Biochemical markers of myocyte injury in heart failure. Heart 2004; 90(10):1110–3.

91. Wallace TW, Abdullah SM, Drazner MH, et al. Prevalence and determinants of troponin T elevation in the general population. Circulation 2006;113(16): 1958–65.

92. Sundstrom J, Ingelsson E, Berglund L, et al. Cardiac troponin-I and risk of heart failure: a community-based cohort study. Eur Heart J 2009;30(7):773–81.

93. Cardinale D, Sandri MT, Colombo A, et al. Prognostic value of troponin I in cardiac risk stratification of cancer patients undergoing high-dose chemotherapy. Circulation 2004;109(22): 2749–54.

94. Cardinale D, Sandri MT, Martinoni A, et al. Left ventricular dysfunction predicted by early troponin I release after high-dose chemotherapy. J Am Coll Cardiol 2000;36(2):517–22.

95. Biolo A, Fisch M, Balog J, et al. Episodes of acute heart failure syndrome are associated with increased levels of troponin and extracellular matrix markers. Circ Heart Fail 2010;3(1):44–50.

96. Weber KT, Sun Y, Tyagi SC, et al. Collagen network of the myocardium: function, structural remodeling and regulatory mechanisms. J Mol Cell Cardiol 1994;26(3):279–92.

97. Gunja-Smith Z, Morales AR, Romanelli R, et al. Remodeling of human myocardial collagen in idiopathic dilated cardiomyopathy. Role of metalloproteinases and pyridinoline cross-links. Am J Pathol 1996; 148(5):1639–48.

98. Rossi MA, Abreu MA, Santoro LB. Images in cardiovascular medicine. Connective tissue skeleton of the human heart: a demonstration by cell-maceration scanning electron microscope method. Circulation 1998;97(9):934–5.

99. Spinale FG, Tomita M, Zellner JL, et al. Collagen remodeling and changes in LV function during development and recovery from supraventricular tachycardia. Am J Physiol 1991;261(2 Pt 2): H308–18.

100. Weber KT, Pick R, Janicki JS, et al. Inadequate collagen tethers in dilated cardiopathy. Am Heart J 1988;116(6 Pt 1):1641–6.

101. Abrahams C, Janicki JS, Weber KT. Myocardial hypertrophy in Macaca fascicularis. Structural remodeling of the collagen matrix. Lab Invest 1987; 56(6):676–83.

102. Weber KT, Janicki JS, Shroff SG, et al. Collagen remodeling of the pressure-overloaded, hypertrophied nonhuman primate myocardium. Circ Res 1988;62(4):757–65.

103. Schaper J, Speiser B. The extracellular matrix in the failing human heart. Basic Res Cardiol 1992; 87(Suppl 1):303–9.

104. Weber KT, Brilla CG. Pathological hypertrophy and cardiac interstitium. Fibrosis and renin-angiotensin-aldosterone system. Circulation 1991; 83(6):1849–65.

105. Kato S, Spinale FG, Tanaka R, et al. Inhibition of collagen cross-linking: effects on fibrillar collagen and ventricular diastolic function. Am J Physiol 1995;269(3 Pt 2):H863–8.

106. Stroud JD, Baicu CF, Barnes MA, et al. Viscoelastic properties of pressure overload hypertrophied myocardium: effect of serine protease treatment. Am J Physiol Heart Circ Physiol 2002;282(6):H2324–35.

107. Katz AM, Zile MR. New molecular mechanism in diastolic heart failure. Circulation 2006;113(16): 1922–5.

108. Zile MR, Baicu CF, Gaasch WH. Diastolic heart failure–abnormalities in active relaxation and passive stiffness of the left ventricle. N Engl J Med 2004;350(19):1953–9.

109. Dell'italia LJ, Balcells E, Meng QC, et al. Volume-overload cardiac hypertrophy is unaffected by ACE inhibitor treatment in dogs. Am J Physiol 1997;273(2 Pt 2):H961–70.

110. Spinale FG, Ishihra K, Zile M, et al. Structural basis for changes in left ventricular function and geometry because of chronic mitral regurgitation and after correction of volume overload. J Thorac Cardiovasc Surg 1993;106(6):1147–57.

111. Weber KT, Pick R, Silver MA, et al. Fibrillar collagen and remodeling of dilated canine left ventricle. Circulation 1990;82(4):1387–401.

112. Spinale FG. Myocardial matrix remodeling and the matrix metalloproteinases: influence on cardiac form and function. Physiol Rev 2007;87(4): 1285–342.

113. Brew K, Dinakarpandian D, Nagase H. Tissue inhibitors of metalloproteinases: evolution, structure and function. Biochim Biophys Acta 2000; 1477(1–2):267–83.

114. Nagase H, Visse R, Murphy G. Structure and function of matrix metalloproteinases and TIMPs. Cardiovasc Res 2006;69(3):562–73.

115. Deschamps AM, Spinale FG. Pathways of matrix metalloproteinase induction in heart failure: bioactive molecules and transcriptional regulation. Cardiovasc Res 2006;69(3):666–76.

116. Sundstrom J, Evans JC, Benjamin EJ, et al. Relations of plasma total TIMP-1 levels to cardiovascular risk factors and echocardiographic measures: the Framingham heart study. Eur Heart J 2004;25(17): 1509–16.

117. Rossi A, Cicoira M, Golia G, et al. Amino-terminal propeptide of type III procollagen is associated with restrictive mitral filling pattern in patients with dilated cardiomyopathy: a possible link between diastolic dysfunction and prognosis. Heart 2004; 90(6):650–4.

118. Mizon-Gerard F, de Groote P, Lamblin N, et al. Prognostic impact of matrix metalloproteinase gene polymorphisms in patients with heart failure according to the aetiology of left ventricular systolic dysfunction. Eur Heart J 2004;25(8):688–93.

119. Kelly D, Cockerill G, Ng LL, et al. Plasma matrix metalloproteinase-9 and left ventricular remodelling after acute myocardial infarction in man: a prospective cohort study. Eur Heart J 2007; 28(6):711–8.

120. Cavusoglu E, Ruwende C, Chopra V, et al. Tissue inhibitor of metalloproteinase-1 (TIMP-1) is an independent predictor of all-cause mortality, cardiac mortality, and myocardial infarction. Am Heart J 2006;151(5):1101.e1–8.

121. Anker SD, von Haehling S. Inflammatory mediators in chronic heart failure: an overview. Heart 2004; 90(4):464–70.

122. Seta Y, Shan K, Bozkurt B, et al. Basic mechanisms in heart failure: the cytokine hypothesis. J Card Fail 1996;2(3):243–9.

123. Elster SK, Braunwald E, Wood HF. A study of C-reactive protein in the serum of patients with congestive heart failure. Am Heart J 1956;51(4): 533–41.

124. Vasan RS, Sullivan LM, Roubenoff R, et al. Inflammatory markers and risk of heart failure in elderly subjects without prior myocardial infarction: the Framingham Heart Study. Circulation 2003; 107(11):1486–91.

125. Cicoira M, Bolger AP, Doehner W, et al. High tumour necrosis factor-alpha levels are associated with exercise intolerance and neurohormonal activation in chronic heart failure patients. Cytokine 2001;15(2):80–6.

126. Deswal A, Petersen NJ, Feldman AM, et al. Cytokines and cytokine receptors in advanced heart failure: an analysis of the cytokine database from the Vesnarinone trial (VEST). Circulation 2001; 103(16):2055–9.

127. Gwechenberger M, Hulsmann M, Berger R, et al. Interleukin-6 and B-type natriuretic peptide are independent predictors for worsening of heart failure in patients with progressive congestive heart failure. J Heart Lung Transplant 2004;23(7):839–44.

128. Tsutamoto T, Hisanaga T, Fukai D, et al. Prognostic value of plasma soluble intercellular adhesion molecule-1 and endothelin-1 concentration in patients with chronic congestive heart failure. Am J Cardiol 1995;76(11):803–8.

129. Yin WH, Chen JW, Young MS, et al. Increased endothelial monocyte adhesiveness is related to clinical outcomes in chronic heart failure. Int J Cardiol 2007;121(3):276–83.

130. Anand IS, Florea VG. Traditional and novel approaches to management of heart failure: successes and failures. Cardiol Clin 2008;26(1): 59–72, vi.

131. Cave AC, Brewer AC, Narayanapanicker A, et al. NADPH oxidases in cardiovascular health and disease. Antioxid Redox Signal 2006;8(5–6):691–728.

132. Ungvari Z, Gupte SA, Recchia FA, et al. Role of oxidative-nitrosative stress and downstream pathways in various forms of cardiomyopathy and heart failure. Curr Vasc Pharmacol 2005;3(3):221–9.

133. Kameda K, Matsunaga T, Abe N, et al. Correlation of oxidative stress with activity of matrix metalloproteinase in patients with coronary artery disease. Possible role for left ventricular remodelling. Eur Heart J 2003;24(24):2180–5.

134. Hokamaki J, Kawano H, Yoshimura M, et al. Urinary biopyrrins levels are elevated in relation to severity of heart failure. J Am Coll Cardiol 2004;43(10): 1880–5.

135. Keith M, Geranmayegan A, Sole MJ, et al. Increased oxidative stress in patients with congestive heart failure. J Am Coll Cardiol 1998;31(6):1352–6.

136. Nonaka-Sarukawa M, Yamamoto K, Aoki H, et al. Increased urinary 15-F2t-isoprostane concentrations in patients with non-ischaemic congestive heart failure: a marker of oxidative stress. Heart 2003;89(8):871–4.

137. Wykretowicz A, Furmaniuk J, Smielecki J, et al. The oxygen stress index and levels of circulating interleukin-10 and interleukin-6 in patients with

chronic heart failure. Int J Cardiol 2004;94(2–3): 283–7.

138. Ferrari R, Guardigli G, Mele D, et al. Oxidative stress during myocardial ischaemia and heart failure. Curr Pharm Des 2004;10(14):1699–711.

139. Pacher P, Schulz R, Liaudet L, et al. Nitrosative stress and pharmacological modulation of heart failure. Trends Pharmacol Sci 2005;26(6):302–10.

140. Berry CE, Hare JM. Xanthine oxidoreductase and cardiovascular disease: molecular mechanisms and pathophysiological implications. J Physiol 2004;555(Pt 3):589–606.

141. Baldus S, Mullerleile K, Chumley P, et al. Inhibition of xanthine oxidase improves myocardial contractility in patients with ischemic cardiomyopathy. Free Radic Biol Med 2006;41(8):1282–8.

142. George J, Carr E, Davies J, et al. High-dose allopurinol improves endothelial function by profoundly reducing vascular oxidative stress and not by lowering uric acid. Circulation 2006;114(23): 2508–16.

143. Kittleson MM, St John ME, Bead V, et al. Increased levels of uric acid predict haemodynamic compromise in patients with heart failure independently of B-type natriuretic peptide levels. Heart 2007;93(3): 365–7.

144. Leyva F, Anker S, Swan JW, et al. Serum uric acid as an index of impaired oxidative metabolism in chronic heart failure. Eur Heart J 1997;18(5): 858–65.

145. Doehner W, Rauchhaus M, Florea VG, et al. Uric acid in cachectic and noncachectic patients with chronic heart failure: relationship to leg vascular resistance. Am Heart J 2001;141(5):792–9.

146. Anker SD, Doehner W, Rauchhaus M, et al. Uric acid and survival in chronic heart failure: validation and application in metabolic, functional, and hemodynamic staging. Circulation 2003;107(15):1991–7.

147. Baldus S, Koster R, Chumley P, et al. Oxypurinol improves coronary and peripheral endothelial function in patients with coronary artery disease. Free Radic Biol Med 2005;39(9):1184–90.

148. Cappola TP, Kass DA, Nelson GS, et al. Allopurinol improves myocardial efficiency in patients with idiopathic dilated cardiomyopathy. Circulation 2001;104(20):2407–11.

149. Cingolani HE, Plastino JA, Escudero EM, et al. The effect of xanthine oxidase inhibition upon ejection fraction in heart failure patients: La Plata Study. J Card Fail 2006;12(7):491–8.

150. Hare JM, Mangal B, Brown J, et al. Impact of oxypurinol in patients with symptomatic heart failure. Results of the OPT-CHF study. J Am Coll Cardiol 2008;51(24):2301–9.

151. Simonet WS, Lacey DL, Dunstan CR, et al. Osteoprotegerin: a novel secreted protein involved in the regulation of bone density. Cell 1997;89(2):309–19.

152. Gupta S, Drazner MH, de Lemos JA. Newer biomarkers in heart failure. Heart Fail Clin 2009; 5(4):579–88.

153. Yun TJ, Chaudhary PM, Shu GL, et al. OPG/FDCR-1, a TNF receptor family member, is expressed in lymphoid cells and is up-regulated by ligating CD40. J Immunol 1998;161(11):6113–21.

154. Ueland T, Yndestad A, Oie E, et al. Dysregulated osteoprotegerin/RANK ligand/RANK axis in clinical and experimental heart failure. Circulation 2005; 111(19):2461–8.

155. Ueland T, Jemtland R, Godang K, et al. Prognostic value of osteoprotegerin in heart failure after acute myocardial infarction. J Am Coll Cardiol 2004; 44(10):1970–6.

156. Omland T, Drazner MH, Ueland T, et al. Plasma osteoprotegerin levels in the general population: relation to indices of left ventricular structure and function. Hypertension 2007;49(6):1392–8.

157. van Kimmenade RR, Januzzi JL Jr, Ellinor PT, et al. Utility of amino-terminal pro-brain natriuretic peptide, galectin-3, and apelin for the evaluation of patients with acute heart failure. J Am Coll Cardiol 2006;48(6):1217–24.

158. Taupenot L, Harper KL, O'Connor DT. The chromogranin-secretogranin family. N Engl J Med 2003;348(12):1134–49.

159. Pieroni M, Corti A, Tota B, et al. Myocardial production of chromogranin A in human heart: a new regulatory peptide of cardiac function. Eur Heart J 2007;28(9):1117–27.

160. Ceconi C, Ferrari R, Bachetti T, et al. Chromogranin A in heart failure; a novel neurohumoral factor and a predictor for mortality. Eur Heart J 2002;23(12): 967–74.

161. Wohlschlaeger J, von Winterfeld M, Milting H, et al. Decreased myocardial chromogranin a expression and colocalization with brain natriuretic peptide during reverse cardiac remodeling after ventricular unloading. J Heart Lung Transplant 2008;27(4): 442–9.

162. Bootcov MR, Bauskin AR, Valenzuela SM, et al. MIC-1, a novel macrophage inhibitory cytokine, is a divergent member of the TGF-beta superfamily. Proc Natl Acad Sci U S A 1997;94(21): 11514–9.

163. Kempf T, von Haehling S, Peter T, et al. Prognostic utility of growth differentiation factor-15 in patients with chronic heart failure. J Am Coll Cardiol 2007; 50(11):1054–60.

164. Arab S, Gramolini AO, Ping P, et al. Cardiovascular proteomics: tools to develop novel biomarkers and potential applications. J Am Coll Cardiol 2006; 48(9):1733–41.

165. Morrow DA, de Lemos JA. Benchmarks for the assessment of novel cardiovascular biomarkers. Circulation 2007;115(8):949–52.

The Role of Renin Angiotensin System Intervention in Stage B Heart Failure

Patrick Collier, MB, PhD, Kenneth M. McDonald, MD*

KEYWORDS

- Heart failure • Left ventricle
- Angiotensin-converting enzyme

The publication of V-HeFT I (Vasodilator-Heart Failure Trial I) in 1985 demonstrated for the first time that the natural history of heart failure (HF) could be beneficially altered by pharmacologic intervention.[1] In the quarter century since that important observation, further significant advances have been made highlighting the growth in the understanding of the HF syndrome that has fostered the development of varied effective pharmacologic and nonpharmacologic approaches to care. Improved prognosis and reduced morbidity have been witnessed predominantly not only with agents that modulate the renin angiotensin aldosterone system (RAAS) and the sympathetic system but also with alternative strategies.

While these advances have been encouraging, the outlook for patients with HF remains a concern. Epidemiologic studies continue to show significant morbidity burden and curtailed life expectancy. Indicative of this is a recent study from Spain in which Gomez-Soto and colleagues,[2] in a large community of HF population, demonstrated that the 4-year mortality for patients with newly diagnosed HF was 61.4%. Furthermore, the advances in HF therapeutics have almost exclusively been confined to patients with reduced left ventricular ejection fraction (LVEF). An increasing proportion of the population has HF with preserved ejection fraction for which the understanding of pathophysiology is poor and whereby therapeutics interventions are, as a result, limited.

Accordingly, increasing emphasis has been placed on the presymptomatic phase of left ventricular (LV) dysfunction. This often prolonged asymptomatic period allows therapeutic interventions to be applied, which may alter the natural history, and prevents or at least delays the evolution to HF. Formal recognition of the importance of this phase of HF came with the American College of Cardiology/American Heart Association guidelines in 2001 in which stages of HF were defined and patients with asymptomatic structural abnormalities of the left ventricle were classified as stage B HF.[3] Those with previous myocardial infarction (MI), LV remodeling including LV hypertrophy (LVH) and low ejection fraction, as well as asymptomatic valvular disease were all included. A better understanding of the predominant pathophysiologic signals at this stage of the HF syndrome may spawn new therapeutic approaches to improve the outlook for patients with ventricular dysfunction. Given that the structural and functional characteristics of stage B HF are relevant to both reduced and preserved ejection faction HF, it is also possible that focusing attention of this phase of HF may allow for

Funding: This work was supported by the Health Research Board of Ireland (RP/2007/313 to K.McD.), Molecular Medicine Ireland (Clinician Scientist Fellowship to P.C.), an unrestricted educational grant from Servier Pharmaceuticals and the MEDIA project (FP7 Health 2010 261409).

Conflict of Interest: K.M.M. has honoraria with Inverness Medical Innovations, Inc.

Heart Failure Unit, St Vincent's University Hospital, Elm Park, Dublin 4, Ireland

* Corresponding author.

E-mail address: kenneth.mcdonald@ucd.ie

a more effective approach to HF with preserved ejection fraction in the future.

As already mentioned, RAAS intervention has been particularly effective in improving the outlook for patients with reduced ejection fraction HF. In addition, there are extensive data linking abnormalities in the RAAS system to the early stages of various forms of cardiomyopathy. Therefore, there is a sound rationale to exploring the benefits of RAAS modulation in stage B HF. This article outlines the link between the RAAS and various forms of cardiomyopathy, and also reviews our understanding of the effectiveness of RAAS intervention in this phase of ventricular dysfunction.

THE ROLE OF RAAS ACTIVATION IN STAGE B HF

The RAAS is a critical component of cardiac neurohormonal signaling and forms the basis of the adaptive homeostatic myocardial response. Most cardiac effects attributed to RAAS activation are mediated by angiotensin II formed after the cleavage effects of angiotensin-converting enzyme (ACE) on angiotensin I, which itself is formed from angiotensinogen by the hormone renin. The heart contains a complete and fully functional RAAS system (including renin, angiotensin, ACE, and angiotensin receptors), and recent evidence suggests that the majority of myocardial angiotensin II is actually derived from local synthesis rather than reuptake from the systemic circulation.[4–6] Non–ACE-dependent pathways to angiotensin II formation also exist in the heart, and together the net result of such local synthetic mechanisms is that the concentration of angiotensin II is typically 100 times higher in cardiac interstitial fluid than in plasma.[7,8] Angiotensin II, by the induction of aldosterone synthase, also enhances the secretion of aldosterone, a cocontributor to cardiac remodeling.[9] Again, aldosterone levels are typically more than 17 times higher in interstitial fluid than in plasma.[10]

In cardiac disease, this signaling pathway is activated excessively and can contribute in a maladaptive fashion to perpetuate disease mechanisms. Given that most of the evidence for the importance of RAAS and the benefits of pharmacologic manipulation of this system has been derived from ischemic, hypertensive, or diabetic cardiomyopathy, the discussion here focuses on patients who have had previous MI or who have LVH. Stage B HF clearly encompasses a wide range of pathologies, and the authors also briefly discuss the role of RAAS activation and intervention in patients with alcoholic cardiomyopathy.

Ischemic Heart Disease (Patients with Previous MI)

In the immediate postinfarction period, RAAS activation occurs as the body attempts to restore hemodynamic balance. However, this comes at a price, and angiotensin II–mediated vasoconstriction together with endothelial dysfunction related to enhanced bradykinin breakdown can further impede coronary blood flow to ischemic regions.[11–13] In addition, myocardial oxygen supply/demand ratios worsen because of RAAS activation through increased superoxide generation and depletion of high-energy phosphate stores.[13,14] Angiotensin II also plays an important role in early remodeling of the infarct zone, and, as a potent inflammatory mediator, it modulates oxidative stress mechanisms, causes increased tissue permeability via increases in vascular endothelial growth factor, and stimulates the release of monocyte chemoattractant protein 1 to activate macrophages and monocytes to move to the site of injury and contribute to wound healing.[15–18] Angiotensin II is also a critical mediator of fibrosis via aldosterone and fibrotic pathways, including transforming growth factor β (TGF-β), connective tissue growth factor, and tissue inhibitor of matrix metalloproteinase (MMP) 1.[19–21]

Activation of the local RAAS by serine proteases in the noninfarcted myocardium means that myocardial tissue remote from the infarct is also not spared the effects of angiotensin II. Upregulation of angiotensinogen gene expression and increased local ACE activity enhances local angiotensin II production, which is the likely stimulus for hypertrophy of noninfarcted myocardium.[22] Direct activation of the sympathetic nervous system eventually causes downregulation of cardiac β_1-adrenergic receptors and impaired inotropic and chronotropic responses, whereas angiotensin II also plays a major role in late postinfarct remodeling by contributing to time-dependent progressive ventricular dilatation, distortion of ventricular shape, mural hypertrophy, recruitment of border-zone myocardium into scar, and deterioration of contractile function.[23,24]

Other effects of angiotensin II include hypercoagulability by direct modulation of levels of tissue plasminogen activator, plasminogen activator inhibitor 1, and tissue factor.[15,25,26] Accumulation of ACE in clustered macrophages and microvessel endothelial cells within human atherosclerotic plaques contributes to increased production of local angiotensin and inflammatory mediators within the vascular wall such as interleukin 6, which together increase the risk of plaque rupture and recurrent MI.[27]

Hypertensive Heart Disease (Patients with LVH)

RAAS activation is a major contributor to the cause and perpetuation of both major structural complications of the left ventricle in hypertensive heart disease (HHD), namely hypertrophy and fibrosis. Inappropriately normal or high renin levels are evident in more than 75% of patients with early hypertension.[28] These levels are typically inappropriate to the systemic hemodynamic milieu of earlier disease phases in which younger patients with hypertension tend to have a high cardiac index/low total peripheral resistance pattern, and one would anticipate plasma renin levels to be low via negative feedback mechanisms.[28,29] Thereafter, an increased level of angiotensin II can promote remodeling by interacting with angiotensin type 1 (AT1) receptors on cardiac myocytes and cardiac fibroblasts to initiate myocyte hypertrophy and increased collagen synthesis, respectively.[30–34] Angiotensin II can also induce cardiac hypertrophy by a novel intracrine mechanism that is independent of AT1.[35]

There is good supportive evidence from animal gene-expression models that hypertrophic factors such as angiotensin II play an important role in such structural changes. For example, transgenic mice overexpressing angiotensinogen develop myocardial hypertrophy independently of hypertension.[36] Equally, transgenic mice with overexpression of the AT1 receptor within cardiac myocytes develop exaggerated cardiac hypertrophy and remodeling, whereas AT1 receptor knockouts show an attenuated hypertrophic and fibrotic response as well as a lower incidence of overt HF compared with wild types.[37,38] Regression analyses in young healthy subjects have shown RAAS activation and, in particular, plasma angiotensin II levels to correlate significantly with LV mass independently of systolic blood pressure.[39] Such hypertrophic signals may coincide or even predate the development of hypertension as evidenced by the fact that LV mass in previously normotensive subjects closely correlates with the subsequent risk of development of hypertension.[40]

An increased likelihood of hypertrophy is seen in patients with more frequent hypertensive daytime recordings during ambulatory monitoring of blood pressure and in those with nocturnal hypertension, higher maximal daytime blood pressures, and peak exercise blood pressures.[41] Such

hemodynamic factors in HHD may exert their hypertrophic responses, although the RAAS as mechanical stretch has been shown to directly increase angiotensin II release from cardiac myocytes.[42]

Hypertrophy and fibrosis underpin LV diastolic dysfunction, a common finding in patients with hypertension. In addition to LVH and fibrosis, maladaptive consequences of prolonged neurohumoral activation in HHD include increased afterload, filling pressures, and heart rate, myocyte apoptosis, and production of fetal isoforms of contractile proteins.

Diabetic Heart Disease (Patients with Previous MI or LVH)

Given the high prevalence of comorbid hypertension and ischemic heart disease in patients with diabetes, much of the previous discussion also applies here. However, this cohort deserves special mention, given that stage B HF is a common finding in patients with diabetes, many of whom have LVH or have had a previous MI. The association of diabetes with hypertension has been shown to accelerate LV diastolic dysfunction mainly through RAAS activation and oxidative stress.[43] Furthermore, in patients with ischemic cardiomyopathy, diabetes mellitus (DM) is a proven risk factor for the progression from asymptomatic LV systolic dysfunction to symptomatic HF.[44] However, diabetes can cause functional, biochemical, and morphologic abnormalities of cardiomyocytes independent of hypertension or coronary disease.[43] Evidence for RAAS activation in the heart of patients with diabetes includes upregulation of cardiac ACE and AT1 receptors, which combine to increase the amount and potency of angiotensin II.[45] Downstream effects then include increased TGF-β activation and formation of reactive oxygen species, both of which strongly promote myocardial fibrosis, a characteristic feature of diabetic heart disease.[46,47]

Toxin-Related Cardiomyopathy (Low Ejection Fraction)

Alcohol is a known myocardial toxin that has been implicated in the causes of cardiomyopathy in circumstances where a history of excess chronic ingestion is documented.[48] Although nutritional deficiencies may contribute, activation of RAAS is also thought to be particularly relevant.[49] Whereas RAAS activation may represent a primary effect of alcohol, alcohol-induced cardiac depression resulting in hemodynamic overload may cause secondary RAAS activation.[50] The markedly divergent impact on the myocardium that can occur between patients despite similar alcohol exposures led many to suspect a genetic susceptibility to alcohol-induced cardiomyopathy. Supportive evidence for this hypothesis was found in a recent study by Fernandez-Sola and colleagues[51] involving ACE gene polymorphisms, previously linked to idiopathic cardiomyopathy and HHD. Patients homozygous for the D allele were 16.4 times more likely to develop alcohol-related cardiac depression. The D allele has been associated with higher circulating levels of ACE and angiotensin II.[52] Furthermore, the DD genotype is associated with more rapid progression to overt HF as well as an increased rate of adverse cardiovascular events.[53]

Another well-described form of toxin-induced cardiomyopathy is that related to anthracycline chemotherapy in the setting of treatment of malignancy. Although many mechanisms may be at play in the production of anthracycline cardiotoxicity, there is evidence that the RAAS system may be involved. In an AT1 receptor knockout mouse model, Toko and colleagues[54] demonstrated that anthracycline therapy induced myofibrillar loss and increased the number of apoptotic cells in wild-type mice, but not in knockout mice. Although downregulated atrial natriuretic peptide gene expression was evident in wild-type mice, this alteration was attenuated in AT1 knockout mice.

RAAS activation also appears to be of relevance in viral and nonviral myocarditis. In an AT1 receptor knockout mouse model, Yamamoto and colleagues[55] demonstrated reduced expression of proinflammatory cytokines in response to viral injury in knockout mice that was associated with an improved survival at 14 days, consistent with the known role of angiotensin II in the inflammatory reaction. Hanawa and colleagues[56] also demonstrated activation of the RAAS in an experimental model of autoimmune myocarditis.

RAAS INTERVENTIONS IN STAGE B HF

For patients with stage B HF, the primary goal of therapy is prevention of overt disease, a vital component of which involves the therapeutic manipulation of the RAAS. ACE inhibitors mediate vasodilation by inhibiting the formation of the potent vasoconstrictor angiotensin II while also limiting degradation of the vasodilator bradykinin. Short-term ACE-inhibitor therapy lowers plasma and tissue angiotensin II. Although angiotensin II typically returns to pretherapeutic levels, due to "escape" via non–ACE-dependent pathways, the benefits of ACE inhibitors are maintained over time, implying that suppression of circulating

angiotensin II does not fully account for all of the therapeutic effects seen.[57] Of note, part of the antihypertensive, antifibrotic, and antithrombotic properties of ACE inhibitors are mediated by the preservation of bradykinin levels, known to stimulate nitric oxide production.[58,59] The development of AT1 angiotensin II receptor blockers was achieved more than 15 years ago to try and ameliorate some of the adverse biochemical problems of ACE inhibitors, including angiotensin II escape, accumulation of kinins, and reduction of signaling through the antiproliferative AT2 receptor.[60–63]

Having laid the groundwork for the importance of RAAS activation in stage B HF, the authors now discuss the important RAAS intervention trials that have predominantly involved the use of ACE inhibitors as well as angiotensin receptor blockers (ARBs) and aldosterone antagonists.

Ischemic Heart Disease

Some of the earliest evidence for the benefit of ACE inhibitors following MI came from rat models in which Pfeffer and colleagues[64] demonstrated that captopril could prevent ventricular dilation and increases in chamber stiffness. Human studies quickly followed and again captopril was shown to be beneficial after infarction by attenuating LV remodeling, reducing filling pressures, and improving exercise tolerance.[65] Another study showed that captopril-treated patients did not manifest shape-dependent objective and subjective measures of reduced functional capacity when compared with control patients.[66]

In addition to afterload reduction, accumulating evidence now suggests that ACE inhibitors are also protective against recurrent myocardial ischemia, endothelial dysfunction, reperfusion injury, tissue inflammation, plaque rupture, and clot formation.[11–18] ACE inhibitors protect against LV dilatation and increased wall stress by limiting the remodeling effects of upregulated ACE levels evident in peri-infarct tissue.[67–69] The risk of sudden death is attenuated by a decrease in sympathetic activity, an improvement in baroreceptor sensitivity, and an enhancement of vagal tone. Greater electrical stability is also achieved via improvements in the arrhythmic substrate as a secondary effect of the reduction in ventricular remodeling and the rate of recurrent MI.[70,71] Although attenuated atherosclerosis with ACE inhibitors is a repeated finding in numerous animal models, whether such therapy can prevent or regress atherosclerosis in humans remains controversial.[72–75] For example, in a substudy of the HOPE (Heart Outcomes Prevention Evaluation) study, ramipril reduced plaque size by 0.008 mm/y compared with placebo, in contrast to the negative outcome of the PART-2 (Prevention of Atherosclerosis with Ramipril-2) study.[76,77]

One of the first studies to show cardiac protection by ACE inhibitors in stage B postinfarct patients was the SAVE (the Survival and Ventricular Enlargement) trial.[78] This study randomized 2231 patients who were 3 to 16 days postinfarct with LVEF less than 40% and no overt signs of HF to treatment with captopril or placebo. After an average of 3.5 years, the captopril group demonstrated a relative reduction in all-cause mortality (19%), cardiovascular death (21%), the risk of recurrent MI (25%), and incidence of severe HF (37%). The SOLVD (Studies of Left Ventricular Dysfunction) prevention trial involved 4228 patients with stage B HF (83% of whom had had an MI more than 30 days from entry) with an LVEF less than 35% who were randomly assigned to enalapril (up to 20 mg once per day) or placebo. Enalapril significantly reduced the incidence of progression to overt HF and the rate of related hospitalizations.[79] At a mean follow-up of just over 3 years, enalapril therapy was associated with a nonsignificant reduction in cardiovascular mortality compared with placebo (14% vs 16%). Follow-up echocardiography revealed that enalapril attenuated progressive increases in LV dilatation and hypertrophy in patients with stage B HF.[80] Further confirmation of the efficacy of ACE inhibitors for such patients followed, including the TRACE (Trandolapril Cardiac Evaluation) study, which enrolled 6676 patients with LV dysfunction after MI and randomized patients to trandolapril or placebo.[81] Mortality and progression to severe HF were reduced in the treatment group, which translated to a 15.3-month prolongation of life expectancy at follow-up 6 years later.[82] Two similar trials that followed included very large numbers of patients, one of which was ISIS-4 (Fourth International Study of Infarct Survival) involving 58,050 patients randomized within 24 hours after infarction to either captopril or placebo for 1 month.[83] Captopril therapy was associated with a significant 7% proportional reduction in 5-week mortality, which persisted at 12 months. In GISSI-3 (Gruppo Italiano per lo Studio della Sopravvivenza nell'infarto Miocardico-3) more than 19,000 patients were randomly assigned, again within 24 hours after infarction, to either lisinopril or placebo for 6 weeks.[84] Here, a 10% relative reduction in a combined outcome measure of mortality and severe ventricular dysfunction was evident at 6 weeks, and persisted for at least as long as 4 years despite discontinuation of the drug after 6 weeks.[85] The mortality benefit with ACE inhibition was primarily seen in patients with diabetes, who comprised about 15% of the study population.

Together, such studies firmly established ACE inhibitors as first-line therapy for patients with asymptomatic LV dysfunction following acute MI. In a large meta-analysis of more than 100,000 patients randomized following acute MI, oral ACE inhibitors were associated with a 7% relative reduction in mortality at 30 days.[86] When put in context, the degree of mortality reductions achieved in these ACE-inhibitor trials are generally greater than those achieved with other therapeutic interventions. This is particularly the case for high-risk patients (those with anterior territory infarcts and with severe LV dysfunction) in whom demonstrated benefits are up to10 times greater again than those achieved in low-risk patients (those with normal LVEF and who have been successfully revascularized). Although there is no evidence that early (within 24 hours) treatment with ACE inhibitors is necessarily better than later therapy, early treatment is generally advised on the basis that mortality is highest in the acute phase of acute MI, and that patients in the larger trials were treated early (albeit after timely and careful observation of their hemodynamic and clinical status and after administration of routinely recommended treatments).

Although the duration of treatment in many of the relevant trials of ACE inhibition after MI was 4 to 6 weeks, guidelines suggest indefinite ACE-inhibitor therapy after MI for most patients.[87] Although many postinfarct patients have other specific indications for such therapy, such as HF, diabetes, vascular disease, hypertension, or chronic kidney disease, for patients at low risk the benefits of long-term therapy should be weighed against the potential burdens (side effects, complicated medical regimens, or financial concerns).[87] Further reassessment of LV function should be considered 4 to 6 months after acute MI.[88] The beneficial effect of ACE inhibition in the early postinfarct setting is likely a class effect, given that randomized trials using other ACE inhibitors, including enalapril, ramipril, trandolapril, and zofenopril, have consistently demonstrated favorable efficacy.[81,89–91] Whether class differences exist remains controversial.[92] One caveat relates to the use of intravenous ACE-inhibitor therapy, which is no longer recommended because of adverse outcomes related to the risk of hypotension that were particularly evident in older patients.[93] Of note, patients with stage B HF with renal impairment should not necessarily be excluded from ACE-inhibitor therapy, as a retrospective cohort study of more than 20,000 patients older than 65 years with MI and impaired LV function demonstrated that administration of an ACE inhibitor was associated with a survival benefit even in patients with serum creatinine concentrations of greater than 3 mg/dL (265 μmol/L).[94]

An important point to consider when reviewing these postinfarct ACE-inhibitor trials is that most (more than 70%) patients enrolled had had sinus tachycardia (ST) elevation infarcts and were treated with either fibrinolytic therapy or no reperfusion.[83,84] Thus, data on the efficacy and safety of these therapies in patients with non–ST-elevation acute coronary syndrome or in patients who had percutaneous coronary intervention for MI are limited.

RAAS intervention using ARBs has been investigated in 2 large randomized trials (OPTIMAAL [Optimal Trial in Myocardial Infarction with the Angiotensin II Antagonist Losartan] and VALIANT [Valsartan in Acute Myocardial Infarction]) in which they were compared with ACE inhibitors in the postinfarct setting in high-risk (anterior territory infarct with/without HF) patients. Of importance, no significant difference in mortality was found between the 2 therapies.[95,96] For this reason, guidelines suggest that ARBs can be considered in patients with acute MI who are intolerant of ACE inhibitors, especially in the setting of LV dysfunction. The VALIANT trial also found that combination therapy (ARBs and ACE inhibitor) in the immediate post-MI setting was associated with a higher risk of side effects that lead to reduction in drug doses and so should not be recommended.

HHD (Patients with LVH)

The first indications that ACE-inhibitor therapy would be beneficial in LVH again came from early rat models of hypertension. Chronic therapy with captopril resulted in marked regression of cardiac hypertrophy and was able to prevent deterioration of cardiac performance in rats with long-standing hypertension and LVH. Substantial reductions in LV mass evident in chronically hypertensive rats treated with chronic captopril therapy were also associated with improvements in electrocardiographic abnormalities.[97,98]

When trialed in human studies the benefits of ACE inhibitors were just as impressive, extending right across the spectrum of HHD from those with LV dysfunction to those with HF.[99] Patients who displayed more marked neurohormonal activation gained the largest survival benefit, as reflected by plasma norepinephrine or angiotensin II levels.[79] In patients with asymptomatic LV dysfunction,

ACE-inhibitor therapy prevents the development of HF and reduces hospitalization and cardiovascular death by preventing progressive LV remodeling and progressive atherosclerosis while also lowering the risk of arrhythmia.[100,101] Even at subpressor doses, ACE inhibitors can prevent and even cause regression of LVH and fibrosis.[102–104] Reductions in LVH have been recorded as early as 2 months after initiation of ACE-inhibitor therapy.[105] These structural improvements are also associated with clear improvements of diastolic function.[106] Given the efficacy of optimal medical therapy and RAAS inhibition to cause regression of remodeling, a small subset of patients with HHD with stage B HF may represent patients who previously had established HF but whose disease regressed. Whether such patients remain at higher risk is currently unclear.

Whether RAAS intervention by blockade of angiotensin receptors is as effective as ACE inhibition has been the subject of multiple large, randomized clinical trials. These data suggest that angiotensin II receptor blockers also possess similar benefits to ACE inhibitors in HHD and provide an alternative option, particularly in view of their more favorable side effect profiles.[107,108] Treatment with angiotensin II receptor blocker was shown to result in regression of LV remodeling, LVH, and fibrosis, and to improve diastology.[109,110] Other benefits include modulation of inflammatory pathways via inhibition of oxidative stress and reduced myocyte apoptosis.[111,112]

Contrary to common assumptions, baseline aldosterone levels are typically low or normal in hypertension and HF.[113,114] In fact, the main ligand of the cardiac mineralocorticoid receptor (MR) may be cortisol rather than aldosterone.[115] MR blockade is associated with an increased risk of hyperkalemia and upstream reflex activation of renin and angiotensin II via negative feedback mechanisms. Nevertheless, as antihypertensive agents MR blockers have a characteristically wide range of efficacy and seem to be of particular use in niche cohorts, such as those with resistant hypertension or low-renin hypertension, and black patients.[116,117] Furthermore, antagonism of MR has anti-inflammatory and antifibrotic effects that may offer end-organ protection.[118] This antifibrotic effect may be even stronger when aldosterone antagonism is combined with ACE inhibition.[119] Increases in markers of inflammation and fibrosis may underlie disease progression in patients with diastolic dysfunction. Aggressive RAAS blockade using aldosterone blockers may offer one solution to attenuation of this process.[120]

An important ongoing debate relates to the relative merits of RAAS inhibition versus non-RAAS methods of lowering blood pressure regarding the effect on LV mass reduction. A large meta-analysis involving 80 double-blind, randomized placebo-controlled trials and more than 4000 patients examined this precise question.[121] After adjustment for duration of treatment and changes in blood pressure, significant differences were seen between drug classes. LV mass index decreased by 13% (8%–18%) with angiotensin II receptor antagonists, by 11% (9%–13%) with calcium antagonists, by 10% (8%–12%) with ACE inhibitors, by 8% (5%–10%) with diuretics, and by 6% (3%–8%) with β-blockers (95% confidence interval shown in parentheses). Pairwise comparison tests revealed that angiotensin II receptor antagonists, calcium antagonists, and ACE inhibitors were more effective at reducing LV mass than were β-blockers (all $P<.05$ with Bonferroni correction).

Diabetic Heart Disease (Patients with Previous MI or LVH)

Patients with hypertensive or ischemic cardiomyopathy who have comorbid diabetes tend to have more marked neurohormonal activation and so derive considerable benefit from ACE inhibitors.[79] RAAS intervention can ameliorate diastolic dysfunction in patients with HHD complicated with DM in humans.[43] Furthermore, the incidence of diabetes in patients with LV dysfunction is significantly reduced by enalapril, especially those with impaired fasting glucose level, while clinical proteinuria, an independent predictor of hospitalization for congestive HF and mortality in patients with diabetes with LV dysfunction, is also significantly reduced.[122,123]

Toxin-Related Cardiomyopathy

The impact of RAAS-modulating therapy was tested in a canine model of alcohol-related cardiomyopathy by Cheng and colleagues.[124] Dogs fed with an alcohol-rich diet had increased circulating and tissue levels of renin and angiotensin II as well as increased intracardiac ACE activity and myocyte AT1 receptor expression. Of importance, this serum and tissue RAAS activation was then followed by a progressive decrease in LV contractility that was associated with abnormalities in myocyte calcium signaling. The angiotensin II receptor blocker irbesartan was found to prevent alcohol-induced decreases in LV and myocyte function and to restore normal myocyte calcium signaling.

RAAS-modulating therapy has also been shown to be of benefit in anthracycline therapy. Cadeddu and colleagues[125] demonstrated that the AT1

> **Box 1**
> **Key Points**
>
> - Evidence for RAAS activation is present in all forms of cardiomyopathy.
> - Underpinning therapeutics for established HF, RAAS interventions also have proven efficacy for those with stage B HF.
> - Focused attention on earlier disease phases may allow for more effective future preventive strategies for patients with HF.

receptor blocker telmisartan prevented the early features of epirubicin-induced cardiomyopathy, again suggesting the importance of the AT1 receptor in anthracycline cardiomyopathy.

Xiao and colleagues[126] showed that eplerenone can beneficially modulate viral myocarditis with less myocardial fibrosis 28 days after inoculation, possibly because of reduced early production of mast cell proteases and MMP-9.

SUMMARY AND FUTURE DIRECTIONS

This review underlines the central role of the RAAS in stage B cardiomyopathy of varied causes. Furthermore, it is clear that similar to stage C and D HF, RAAS therapy is very effective at modulating the natural history of many forms of asymptomatic LV dysfunction. These observations underline the importance of identifying stage B HF, a process that requires implementation of an effective screening strategy.

Although much has been achieved with RAAS-modulating therapy in this phase of HF, many questions remain to be resolved. In particular, attention needs to be directed toward asymptomatic LV diastolic dysfunction, a common finding in stage B HF known to influence prognosis, in which the benefits of RAAS modulation are as yet unknown. **Box 1** summarizes the key points of this article.

REFERENCES

1. Cohn JN, Archibald DG, Ziesche S, et al. Effect of vasodilator therapy on mortality in chronic congestive heart failure. Results of a Veterans Administration Cooperative Study. N Engl J Med 1986; 314(24):1547–52.
2. Gomez-Soto FM, Andrey JL, Garcia-Egido AA, et al. Incidence and mortality of heart failure: a community-based study. Int J Cardiol 2011; 151(1):40–5.
3. Hunt SA, Abraham WT, Chin MH, et al. ACC/AHA 2005 Guideline Update for the Diagnosis and

Management of Chronic Heart Failure in the Adult: a report of the American College of Cardiology/ American Heart Association Task Force on Practice Guidelines (Writing Committee to Update the 2001 Guidelines for the Evaluation and Management of Heart Failure): developed in collaboration with the American College of Chest Physicians and the International Society for Heart and Lung Transplantation: endorsed by the Heart Rhythm Society. Circulation 2005;112(12):e154–235.

4. Danser AH, van Kats JP, Admiraal PJ, et al. Cardiac renin and angiotensins. Uptake from plasma versus in situ synthesis. Hypertension 1994;24(1):37–48.

5. Dell'Italia LJ, Meng QC, Balcells E, et al. Compartmentalization of angiotensin II generation in the dog heart. Evidence for independent mechanisms in intravascular and interstitial spaces. J Clin Invest 1997;100(2):253–8.

6. Dostal DE, Baker KM. The cardiac renin-angiotensin system: conceptual, or a regulator of cardiac function? Circ Res 1999;85(7):643–50.

7. Balcells E, Meng QC, Johnson WH Jr, et al. Angiotensin II formation from ACE and chymase in human and animal hearts: methods and species considerations. Am J Physiol 1997;273(4 Pt 2): H1769–74.

8. Dostal DE. The cardiac renin-angiotensin system: novel signaling mechanisms related to cardiac growth and function. Regul Pept 2000;91(1–3):1–11.

9. Hayashi M, Tsutamoto T, Wada A, et al. Relationship between transcardiac extraction of aldosterone and left ventricular remodeling in patients with first acute myocardial infarction: extracting aldosterone through the heart promotes ventricular remodeling after acute myocardial infarction. J Am Coll Cardiol 2001;38(5):1375–82.

10. Sun Y, Cleutjens JP, Diaz-Arias AA, et al. Cardiac angiotensin converting enzyme and myocardial fibrosis in the rat. Cardiovasc Res 1994;28(9): 1423–32.

11. Schneider CA, Voth E, Moka D, et al. Improvement of myocardial blood flow to ischemic regions by angiotensin-converting enzyme inhibition with quinaprilat IV: a study using [^{15}O] water dobutamine stress positron emission tomography. J Am Coll Cardiol 1999;34(4):1005–11.

12. Li K, Chen X. Protective effects of captopril and enalapril on myocardial ischemia and reperfusion damage of rat. J Mol Cell Cardiol 1987;19(9): 909–15.

13. Mancini GB, Henry GC, Macaya C, et al. Angiotensin-converting enzyme inhibition with quinapril improves endothelial vasomotor dysfunction in patients with coronary artery disease. The TREND (Trial on Reversing Endothelial Dysfunction) Study. Circulation 1996;94(3):258–65.

14. Piana RN, Wang SY, Friedman M, et al. Angiotensin-converting enzyme inhibition preserves endothelium-dependent coronary microvascular responses during short-term ischemia-reperfusion. Circulation 1996;93(3):544–51.

15. Soejima H, Ogawa H, Yasue H, et al. Angiotensin-converting enzyme inhibition reduces monocyte chemoattractant protein-1 and tissue factor levels in patients with myocardial infarction. J Am Coll Cardiol 1999;34(4):983–8.

16. Suzuki Y, Ruiz-Ortega M, Lorenzo O, et al. Inflammation and angiotensin II. Int J Biochem Cell Biol 2003;35(6):881–900.

17. Williams B, Baker AQ, Gallacher B, et al. Angiotensin II increases vascular permeability factor gene expression by human vascular smooth muscle cells. Hypertension 1995;25(5):913–7.

18. Ruiz-Ortega M, Lorenzo O, Suzuki Y, et al. Proinflammatory actions of angiotensins. Curr Opin Nephrol Hypertens 2001;10(3):321–9.

19. Sarkar S, Vellaichamy E, Young D, et al. Influence of cytokines and growth factors in ANG II-mediated collagen upregulation by fibroblasts in rats: role of myocytes. Am J Physiol Heart Circ Physiol 2004;287(1):H107–17.

20. Ruperez M, Lorenzo O, Blanco-Colio LM, et al. Connective tissue growth factor is a mediator of angiotensin II-induced fibrosis. Circulation 2003; 108(12):1499–505.

21. Castoldi G, Di Gioia CR, Pieruzzi F, et al. ANG II increases TIMP-1 expression in rat aortic smooth muscle cells in vivo. Am J Physiol Heart Circ Physiol 2003;284(2):H635–43.

22. Lindpaintner K, Lu W, Neidermajer N, et al. Selective activation of cardiac angiotensinogen gene expression in post-infarction ventricular remodeling in the rat. J Mol Cell Cardiol 1993;25(2):133–43.

23. Nozawa T, Igawa A, Yoshida N, et al. Dual-tracer assessment of coupling between cardiac sympathetic neuronal function and downregulation of beta-receptors during development of hypertensive heart failure of rats. Circulation 1998;97(23): 2359–67.

24. Sutton MG, Sharpe N. Left ventricular remodeling after myocardial infarction: pathophysiology and therapy. Circulation 2000;101(25):2981–8.

25. Vaughan DE, Rouleau JL, Ridker PM, et al. Effects of ramipril on plasma fibrinolytic balance in patients with acute anterior myocardial infarction. HEART Study Investigators. Circulation 1997;96(2):442–7.

26. Minai K, Matsumoto T, Horie H, et al. Bradykinin stimulates the release of tissue plasminogen activator in human coronary circulation: effects of angiotensin-converting enzyme inhibitors. J Am Coll Cardiol 2001;37(6):1565–70.

27. Schieffer B, Schieffer E, Hilfiker-Kleiner D, et al. Expression of angiotensin II and interleukin 6 in

human coronary atherosclerotic plaques: potential
implications for inflammation and plaque instability.
Circulation 2000;101(12):1372–8.

28. Brunner HR, Sealey JE, Laragh JH. Renin
subgroups in essential hypertension. Further analysis of their pathophysiological and epidemiological
characteristics. Circ Res 1973;32(Suppl 1):99–105.

29. Lund-Johansen P. Central haemodynamics in
essential hypertension at rest and during exercise:
a 20-year follow-up study. J Hypertens Suppl 1989;
7(6):S52–5.

30. Matsusaka T, Katori H, Inagami T, et al. Communi-
cation between myocytes and fibroblasts in
cardiac remodeling in angiotensin chimeric mice.
J Clin Invest 1999;103(10):1451–8.

31. Hafizi S, Wharton J, Morgan K, et al. Expression of
functional angiotensin-converting enzyme and AT1
receptors in cultured human cardiac fibroblasts.
Circulation 1998;98(23):2553–9.

32. McEwan PE, Gray GA, Sherry L, et al. Differential
effects of angiotensin II on cardiac cell proliferation
and intramyocardial perivascular fibrosis in vivo.
Circulation 1998;98(24):2765–73.

33. Kawano H, Do YS, Kawano Y, et al. Angiotensin II
has multiple profibrotic effects in human cardiac
fibroblasts. Circulation 2000;101(10):1130–7.

34. Sadoshima J, Izumo S. Molecular characterization
of angiotensin II-induced hypertrophy of cardiac
myocytes and hyperplasia of cardiac fibroblasts.
Critical role of the AT1 receptor subtype. Circ Res
1993;73(3):413–23.

35. Baker KM, Chernin MI, Schreiber T, et al. Evidence
of a novel intracrine mechanism in angiotensin II-
induced cardiac hypertrophy. Regul Pept 2004;
120(1–3):5–13.

36. Mazzolai L, Nussberger J, Aubert JF, et al. Blood
pressure-independent cardiac hypertrophy induced
by locally activated renin-angiotensin system. Hypertension 1998;31(6):1324–30.

37. Paradis P, Dali-Youcef N, Paradis FW, et al. Overexpression of angiotensin II type I receptor in cardiomyocytes induces cardiac hypertrophy and
remodeling. Proc Natl Acad Sci U S A 2000;
97(2):931–6.

38. Harada K, Sugaya T, Murakami K, et al. Angiotensin II type 1A receptor knockout mice display
less left ventricular remodeling and improved
survival after myocardial infarction. Circulation
1999;100(20):2093–9.

39. Harrap SB, Dominiczak AF, Fraser R, et al. Plasma
angiotensin II, predisposition to hypertension, and
left ventricular size in healthy young adults. Circulation 1996;93(6):1148–54.

40. Post WS, Larson MG, Levy D. Impact of left ventricular structure on the incidence of hypertension. The
Framingham Heart Study. Circulation 1994;90(1):
179–85.

41. Pickering TG, Harshfield GA, Devereux RB,
et al. What is the role of ambulatory blood
pressure monitoring in the management of
hypertensive patients? Hypertension 1985;7(2):
171–7.

42. Sadoshima J, Xu Y, Slayter HS, et al. Autocrine
release of angiotensin II mediates stretch-induced
hypertrophy of cardiac myocytes in vitro. Cell
1993;75(5):977–84.

43. Fukui S, Fukumoto Y, Suzuki J, et al. Diabetes mellitus accelerates left ventricular diastolic dysfunction through activation of the renin-angiotensin
system in hypertensive rats. Hypertens Res 2009;
32(6):472–80.

44. Das SR, Drazner MH, Yancy CW, et al. Effects of
diabetes mellitus and ischemic heart disease on
the progression from asymptomatic left ventricular
dysfunction to symptomatic heart failure: a retrospective analysis from the Studies of Left Ventricular Dysfunction (SOLVD) Prevention trial. Am
Heart J 2004;148(5):883–8.

45. Fiordaliso F, Li B, Latini R, et al. Myocyte death
in streptozotocin-induced diabetes in rats in
angiotensin II- dependent. Lab Invest 2000;80(4):
513–27.

46. Weber KT. Extracellular matrix remodeling in heart
failure: a role for de novo angiotensin II generation.
Circulation 1997;96(11):4065–82.

47. Bendall JK, Cave AC, Heymes C, et al. Pivotal role
of a gp91(phox)-containing NADPH oxidase in
angiotensin II-induced cardiac hypertrophy in
mice. Circulation 2002;105(3):293–6.

48. Piano MR. Alcoholic cardiomyopathy: incidence,
clinical characteristics, and pathophysiology. Chest
2002;121(5):1638–50.

49. Kim SD, Beck J, Bieniarz T, et al. A rodent model of
alcoholic heart muscle disease and its evaluation
by echocardiography. Alcohol Clin Exp Res 2001;
25(3):457–63.

50. Collins GB, Brosnihan KB, Zuti RA, et al. Neuroendocrine, fluid balance, and thirst responses to
alcohol in alcoholics. Alcohol Clin Exp Res 1992;
16(2):228–33.

51. Fernandez-Sola J, Nicolas JM, Oriola J, et al.
Angiotensin-converting enzyme gene polymorphism is associated with vulnerability to
lcoholic cardiomyopathy. Ann Intern Med 2002;
137(5 Part 1):321–6.

52. Danser AH, Schalekamp MA, Bax WA, et al. Angio-
tensin-converting enzyme in the human heart.
Effect of the deletion/insertion polymorphism.
Circulation 1995;92(6):1387–8.

53. Bedi MS, Postava LA, Murali S, et al. Interaction of
implantable defibrillator therapy with angiotensin-
converting enzyme deletion/insertion polymorphism. J Cardiovasc Electrophysiol 2004;15(10):
1162–6.

54. Toko H, Oka T, Zou Y, et al. Angiotensin II type 1a receptor mediates doxorubicin-induced cardiomyopathy. Hypertens Res 2002;25(4):597–603.

55. Yamamoto K, Shioi T, Uchiyama K, et al. Attenuation of virus-induced myocardial injury by inhibition of the angiotensin II type 1 receptor signal and decreased nuclear factor-kappa B activation in knockout mice. J Am Coll Cardiol 2003;42(11): 2000–6.

56. Hanawa H, Abe S, Hayashi M, et al. Time course of gene expression in rat experimental autoimmune myocarditis. Clin Sci (Lond) 2002;103(6):623–32.

57. Brown NJ, Vaughan DE. Angiotensin-converting enzyme inhibitors. Circulation 1998;97(14):1411–20.

58. Hornig B, Kohler C, Drexler H. Role of bradykinin in mediating vascular effects of angiotensin-converting enzyme inhibitors in humans. Circulation 1997;95(5):1115–8.

59. Pretorius M, Rosenbaum D, Vaughan DE, et al. Angiotensin-converting enzyme inhibition increases human vascular tissue-type plasminogen activator release through endogenous bradykinin. Circulation 2003;107(4):579–85.

60. Burnier M, Brunner HR. Angiotensin II receptor antagonists. Lancet 2000;355(9204):637–45.

61. Israili ZH, Hall WD. Cough and angioneurotic edema associated with angiotensin-converting enzyme inhibitor therapy. A review of the literature and pathophysiology. Ann Intern Med 1992; 117(3):234–42.

62. Munzenmaier DH, Greene AS. Opposing actions of angiotensin II on microvascular growth and arterial blood pressure. Hypertension 1996;27(3 Pt 2): 760–5.

63. Oliverio MI, Coffman TM. Angiotensin-II-receptors: new targets for antihypertensive therapy. Clin Cardiol 1997;20(1):3–6.

64. Pfeffer JM, Pfeffer MA, Braunwald E. Influence of chronic captopril therapy on the infarcted left ventricle of the rat. Circ Res 1985;57(1):84–95.

65. Pfeffer MA, Lamas GA, Vaughan DE, et al. Effect of captopril on progressive ventricular dilatation after anterior myocardial infarction. N Engl J Med 1988; 319(2):80–6.

66. Lamas GA, Vaughan DE, Parisi AF, et al. Effects of left ventricular shape and captopril therapy on exercise capacity after anterior wall acute myocardial infarction. Am J Cardiol 1989;63(17): 1167–73.

67. Hokimoto S, Yasue H, Fujimoto K, et al. Expression of angiotensin-converting enzyme in remaining viable myocytes of human ventricles after myocardial infarction. Circulation 1996;94(7):1513–8.

68. Oosterga M, Voors AA, de Kam PJ, et al. Plasma angiotensin-converting enzyme activity and left ventricular dilation after myocardial infarction. Circulation 1997;95(12):2607–9.

69. Yousef ZR, Redwood SR, Marber MS. Postinfarction left ventricular remodelling: where are the theories and trials leading us? Heart 2000;83(1):76–80.

70. Domanski MJ, Exner DV, Borkowf CB, et al. Effect of angiotensin converting enzyme inhibition on sudden cardiac death in patients following acute myocardial infarction. A meta-analysis of randomized clinical trials. J Am Coll Cardiol 1999;33(3): 598–604.

71. Hikosaka M, Yuasa F, Yuyama R, et al. Effect of angiotensin-converting enzyme inhibitor on cardiopulmonary baroreflex sensitivity in patients with acute myocardial infarction. Am J Cardiol 2000; 86(11):1241–4, A6.

72. Brasier AR, Recinos A 3rd, Eledrisi MS. Vascular inflammation and the renin-angiotensin system. Arterioscler Thromb Vasc Biol 2002;22(8):1257–66.

73. Hernandez A, Barberi L, Ballerio R, et al. Delapril slows the progression of atherosclerosis and maintains endothelial function in cholesterol-fed rabbits. Atherosclerosis 1998;137(1):71–6.

74. Hayek T, Attias J, Smith J, et al. Antiatherosclerotic and antioxidative effects of captopril in apolipoprotein E-deficient mice. J Cardiovasc Pharmacol 1998;31(4):540–4.

75. Hayek T, Attias J, Coleman R, et al. The angiotensin-converting enzyme inhibitor, fosinopril, and the angiotensin II receptor antagonist, losartan, inhibit LDL oxidation and attenuate atherosclerosis independent of lowering blood pressure in apolipoprotein E deficient mice. Cardiovasc Res 1999;44(3):579–87.

76. Lonn E, Yusuf S, Dzavik V, et al. Effects of ramipril and vitamin E on atherosclerosis: the study to evaluate carotid ultrasound changes in patients treated with ramipril and vitamin E (SECURE). Circulation 2001;103(7):919–25.

77. MacMahon S, Sharpe N, Gamble G, et al. Randomized, placebo-controlled trial of the angiotensin-converting enzyme inhibitor, ramipril, in patients with coronary or other occlusive arterial disease. PART-2 Collaborative Research Group. Prevention of atherosclerosis with ramipril. J Am Coll Cardiol 2000;36(2):438–43.

78. Pfeffer MA, Braunwald E, Moye LA, et al. Effect of captopril on mortality and morbidity in patients with left ventricular dysfunction after myocardial infarction. Results of the survival and ventricular enlargement trial. The SAVE Investigators. N Engl J Med 1992;327(10):669–77.

79. Effect of enalapril on mortality and the development of heart failure in asymptomatic patients with reduced left ventricular ejection fractions. The SOLVD Investigators. N Engl J Med 1992; 327(10):685–91.

80. Greenberg B, Quinones MA, Koilpillai C, et al. Effects of long-term enalapril therapy on cardiac

structure and function in patients with left ventricular dysfunction. Results of the SOLVD echocardiography substudy. Circulation 1995;91(10):2573–81.

81. Kober L, Torp-Pedersen C, Carlsen JE, et al. A clinical trial of the angiotensin-converting-enzyme inhibitor trandolapril in patients with left ventricular dysfunction after myocardial infarction. Trandolapril Cardiac Evaluation (TRACE) Study Group. N Engl J Med 1995;333(25):1670–6.

82. Torp-Pedersen C, Kober L. Effect of ACE inhibitor trandolapril on life expectancy of patients with reduced left-ventricular function after acute myocardial infarction. TRACE Study Group. Trandolapril cardiac evaluation. Lancet 1999;354(9172):9–12.

83. ISIS-4: a randomised factorial trial assessing early oral captopril, oral mononitrate, and intravenous magnesium sulphate in 58,050 patients with suspected acute myocardial infarction. ISIS-4 (Fourth International Study of Infarct Survival) Collaborative Group. Lancet 1995;345(8951):669–85.

84. GISSI-3: effects of lisinopril and transdermal glyceryl trinitrate singly and together on 6-week mortality and ventricular function after acute myocardial infarction. Gruppo Italiano per lo Studio della Sopravvivenza nell'infarto Miocardico. Lancet 1994;343(8906):1115–22.

85. Ferguson JJ. Meeting highlights. Highlights of the 20th congress of the European Society of Cardiology. Circulation 1999;99(9):1127–31.

86. Indications for ACE inhibitors in the early treatment of acute myocardial infarction: systematic overview of individual data from 100,000 patients in randomized trials. ACE Inhibitor Myocardial Infarction Collaborative Group. Circulation 1998;97(22):2202–12.

87. Antman EM, Hand M, Armstrong PW, et al. 2007 focused update of the ACC/AHA 2004 guidelines for the management of patients with ST-elevation myocardial infarction: a report of the American College of Cardiology/American Heart Association Task Force on Practice Guidelines. J Am Coll Cardiol 2008;51(2):210–47.

88. Latini R, Maggioni AP, Flather M, et al. ACE inhibitor use in patients with myocardial infarction. Summary of evidence from clinical trials. Circulation 1995;92(10):3132–7.

89. Schulman SP, Weiss JL, Becker LC, et al. Effect of early enalapril therapy on left ventricular function and structure in acute myocardial infarction. Am J Cardiol 1995;76(11):764–70.

90. Effect of ramipril on mortality and morbidity of survivors of acute myocardial infarction with clinical evidence of heart failure. The Acute Infarction Ramipril Efficacy (AIRE) Study Investigators. Lancet 1993;342(8875):821–8.

91. Ambrosioni E, Borghi C, Magnani B. The effect of the angiotensin-converting-enzyme inhibitor zofenopril on mortality and morbidity after anterior myocardial infarction. The Survival of Myocardial Infarction Long-Term Evaluation (SMILE) Study Investigators. N Engl J Med 1995;332(2):80–5.

92. Hennessy S, Kimmel SE. Is improved survival a class effect of angiotensin-converting enzyme inhibitors? Ann Intern Med 2004;141(2):157–8.

93. Effects of enalapril on mortality in severe congestive heart failure. Results of the Cooperative North Scandinavian Enalapril Survival Study (CONSENSUS). The CONSENSUS Trial Study Group. N Engl J Med 1987;316(23):1429–35.

94. Frances CD, Noguchi H, Massie BM, et al. Are we inhibited? Renal insufficiency should not preclude the use of ACE inhibitors for patients with myocardial infarction and depressed left ventricular function. Arch Intern Med 2000;160(17):2645–50.

95. Dickstein K, Kjekshus J. Effects of losartan and captopril on mortality and morbidity in high-risk patients after acute myocardial infarction: the OPTIMAAL randomised trial. Optimal Trial in Myocardial Infarction with Angiotensin II Antagonist Losartan. Lancet 2002;360(9335):752–60.

96. Pfeffer MA, McMurray JJ, Velazquez EJ, et al. Valsartan, captopril, or both in myocardial infarction complicated by heart failure, left ventricular dysfunction, or both. N Engl J Med 2003;349(20):1893–906.

97. Pfeffer JM, Pfeffer MA, Mirsky I, et al. Regression of left ventricular hypertrophy and prevention of left ventricular dysfunction by captopril in the-spontaneously hypertensive rat. Proc Natl Acad Sci U S A 1982;79(10):3310–4.

98. Kleber FX, Pfeffer MA, Pfeffer JM. Alterations in the electrocardiogram of spontaneously hypertensive rats by chronic antihypertensive therapy with captopril. Clin Exp Hypertens A 1982;4(6):977–87.

99. Flather MD, Yusuf S, Kober L, et al. Long-term ACE-inhibitor therapy in patients with heart failure or left-ventricular dysfunction: a systematic overview of data from individual patients. ACE-Inhibitor Myocardial Infarction Collaborative Group. Lancet 2000;355(9215):1575–81.

100. Yusuf S, Sleight P, Pogue J, et al. Effects of an angiotensin-converting-enzyme inhibitor, ramipril, on cardiovascular events in high-risk patients. The Heart Outcomes Prevention Evaluation Study Investigators. N Engl J Med 2000;342(3):145–53.

101. Fox KM. Efficacy of perindopril in reduction of cardiovascular events among patients with stable coronary artery disease: randomised, double-blind, placebo-controlled, multicentre trial (the EUROPA study). Lancet 2003;362(9386):782–8.

102. Linz W, Jessen T, Becker RH, et al. Long-term ACE inhibition doubles lifespan of hypertensive rats. Circulation 1997;96(9):3164–72.

103. Lonn EM, Yusuf S, Jha P, et al. Emerging role of angiotensin-converting enzyme inhibitors in cardiac and vascular protection. Circulation 1994; 90(4):2056–69.

104. Pahor M, Bernabei R, Sgadari A, et al. Enalapril prevents cardiac fibrosis and arrhythmias in hypertensive rats. Hypertension 1991;18(2):148–57.

105. Sonnenblick EH. Perindopril treatment for congestive heart failure. Am J Cardiol 2001;88(7A): 19i–27i.

106. Brilla CG, Funck RC, Rupp H. Lisinopril-mediated regression of myocardial fibrosis in patients with hypertensive heart disease. Circulation 2000; 102(12):1388–93.

107. Dahlof B, Devereux RB, Kjeldsen SE, et al. Cardiovascular morbidity and mortality in the Losartan Intervention For Endpoint Reduction in Hypertension Study (LIFE): a randomised trial against atenolol. Lancet 2002;359(9311): 995–1003.

108. Yusuf S, Pfeffer MA, Swedberg K, et al. Effects of candesartan in patients with chronic heart failure and preserved left-ventricular ejection fraction: the CHARM-Preserved Trial. Lancet 2003;362(9386): 777–81.

109. Diez J, Querejeta R, Lopez B, et al. Losartan-dependent regression of myocardial fibrosis is associated with reduction of left ventricular chamber stiffness in hypertensive patients. Circulation 2002;105(21):2512–7.

110. Varo N, Iraburu MJ, Varela M, et al. Chronic AT(1) blockade stimulates extracellular collagen type I degradation and reverses myocardial fibrosis in spontaneously hypertensive rats. Hypertension 2000;35(6):1197–202.

111. Fortuno A, Bidegain J, Robador PA, et al. Losartan metabolite EXP3179 blocks NADPH oxidase-mediated superoxide production by inhibiting protein kinase C: potential clinical implications in hypertension. Hypertension 2009;54(4):744–50.

112. Gonzalez A, Lopez B, Ravassa S, et al. Stimulation of cardiac apoptosis in essential hypertension: potential role of angiotensin II. Hypertension 2002;39(1):75–80.

113. Pitt B, Remme W, Zannad F, et al. Eplerenone, a selective aldosterone blocker, in patients with left ventricular dysfunction after myocardial infarction. N Engl J Med 2003;348(14):1309–21.

114. Pitt B, Zannad F, Remme WJ, et al. The effect of spironolactone on morbidity and mortality in patients with severe heart failure. Randomized Aldactone Evaluation Study Investigators. N Engl J Med 1999;341(10):709–17.

115. Funder JW. Mineralocorticoid receptors and cardiovascular damage: it's not just aldosterone. Hypertension 2006;47(4):634–5.

116. Levy DG, Rocha R, Funder JW. Distinguishing the antihypertensive and electrolyte effects of eplerenone. J Clin Endocrinol Metab 2004;89(6):2736–40.

117. Flack JM, Oparil S, Pratt JH, et al. Efficacy and tolerability of eplerenone and losartan in hypertensive black and white patients. J Am Coll Cardiol 2003;41(7):1148–55.

118. Young M, Funder JW. Eplerenone, but not steroid withdrawal, reverses cardiac fibrosis in deoxycorticosterone/salt-treated rats. Endocrinology 2004;145(7):3153–7.

119. Pitt B, Reichek N, Willenbrock R, et al. Effects of eplerenone, enalapril, and eplerenone/enalapril in patients with essential hypertension and left ventricular hypertrophy: the 4E-left ventricular hypertrophy study. Circulation 2003;108(15): 1831–8.

120. Mak GJ, Ledwidge MT, Watson CJ, et al. Natural history of markers of collagen turnover in patients with early diastolic dysfunction and impact of eplerenone. J Am Coll Cardiol 2009;54(18):1674–82.

121. Klingbeil AU, Schneider M, Martus P, et al. A meta-analysis of the effects of treatment on left ventricular mass in essential hypertension. Am J Med 2003;115(1):41–6.

122. Vermes E, Ducharme A, Bourassa MG, et al. Enalapril reduces the incidence of diabetes in patients with chronic heart failure: insight from the Studies Of Left Ventricular Dysfunction (SOLVD). Circulation 2003;107(9):1291–6.

123. Capes SE, Gerstein HC, Negassa A, et al. Enalapril prevents clinical proteinuria in diabetic patients with low ejection fraction. Diabetes Care 2000; 23(3):377–80.

124. Cheng CP, Cheng HJ, Cunningham C, et al. Angiotensin II type 1 receptor blockade prevents alcoholic cardiomyopathy. Circulation 2006;114(3): 226–36.

125. Cadeddu C, Piras A, Mantovani G, et al. Protective effects of the angiotensin II receptor blocker telmisartan on epirubicin-induced inflammation, oxidative stress, and early ventricular impairment. Am Heart J 2010;160(3):487.e1–7.

126. Xiao J, Shimada M, Liu W, et al. Anti-inflammatory effects of eplerenone on viral myocarditis. Eur J Heart Fail 2009;11(4):349–53.

β-Blockers in Stage B: A Precursor of Heart Failure

Mohammad Sarraf, MD, Gary S. Francis, MD*

KEYWORDS

• β-blockers • Heart failure • Stage B • Left ventricle

It is now clear that many patients with heart failure (HF) progressively pass through various stages of structural and functional abnormalities before advanced signs and symptoms emerge.[1] The transition through these stages is poorly understood. In fact, we know more about the treatment of various stages of HF than we do about the underlying biology. For example, it is seemingly clear that β-adrenergic blocking agents mitigate the progression of HF and have powerful antiremodeling properties, but the mechanistic underpinnings whereby this occurs is not clearly understood. It is possible that left ventricular (LV) dysfunction, LV dilation, and other structural geometric changes can reverse back toward normal when β-blockers are used.[2] But how does this occur? Similar improvement in abnormal LV structure and function can occur with the use of renin-angiotensin-aldosterone system (RAAS) blocking agents, including angiotensin-converting enzyme (ACE) inhibitors, angiotensin-receptor blockers (ARBs), and aldosterone receptor blockers.[3,4] The mechanism of how these RAAS blockers improve HF, as with β-blockers, is not entirely clear. Despite consistent improvement in survival demonstrated by numerous and sometimes stunningly positive clinical trials, reversal of the remodeled LV back toward normal does not occur in all patients. Of the 4 major classes of pharmacologic therapy used to treat HF, is there any advantage of β-adrenergic blockers over RAAS blockers or vice versa? These 2 classes of drugs seem to have similar safety and efficacy. It is true that patients with markedly dilated LV who demonstrate extensive LV scar and fibrosis are less likely to have reverse remodeling. Individual patients sometimes do not tolerate these drugs, except perhaps in low doses. It has been the authors' experience that of the 4 classes of drugs described earlier, β-blockers may be associated with the most consistent improvement in ejection fraction (EF).[5] However, there are no comparator clinical trial data to support this observation, and a clinical trial comparing broad classes of treatment will not be forthcoming. This article attempts to summarize the authors' thoughts regarding the use of β-blockers in patients with stage B, a condition known to be a risk factor for the development of HF. Stage B is typically accompanied by structural and functional changes in the LV despite the absence or paucity of symptoms.

ACTIVATION OF NEUROHORMONES IN HF

HF is a progressive clinical syndrome that is initiated by changes in the structure and function of the LV. It has a myriad of causes. Virtually any form of heart disease can lead to the syndrome of HF. The phenotype of HF occurs as a result of changes in myocardial structure or geometry. These changes may occur through mutations; direct injury to the heart, such as acute myocardial infarction; toxic injury to the heart as a result of chemotherapeutic agents, various other drugs, or radiation exposure; intense and persistent activation of the sympathetic nervous system (eg, pheochromocytoma); perverse loading conditions as found in valvular heart disease or hypertension; infections (particular viral infections leading to myocarditis); autoimmune attacks on the heart

Division of Cardiovascular Diseases, University of Minnesota, Room 206, Variety Club Research Center, 420 Delaware Street Southeast, Mayo Mail Code 508, Minneapolis, MN 55455, USA
* Corresponding author.
E-mail address: franc354@umn.edu

Heart Failure Clin 8 (2012) 237–245
doi:10.1016/j.hfc.2012.01.001

muscle and its matrix; and various other forms of injury. Essentially, the development of HF is a response to injury or mutations and it is, therefore, locked into ancient evolutionary *compensatory* mechanism that occurs in response to the injury. Although these so-called compensatory mechanisms are designed to repair the damaged heart or sustain the circulation during a physiologic threat, such as inadequate perfusion to periphery, the compensatory mechanisms can lead to additional cardiac and vascular structural changes that do not necessarily favor survival. Such changes include myocardial fibrosis, LV dilation, heightened systemic vascular resistance, and myocyte growth and proliferation.[6] This so-called remodeling process is caused by many factors, including increased wall stress, neurohormones, and various cytokines. However, a fundamental driving force is the activation of neurohormonal systems. It is these so-called compensatory neurohormonal systems that antiremodeling agents, including β-blockers, ACE inhibitors, ARBs, and aldosterone receptor blockers, are designed to offset.

HALLMARKS OF HF

LV dysfunction activates many compensatory mechanisms, including release of renin, enhanced exocytosis of norepinephrine (NE) from sympathetic neurons, and heightened arginine vasopressin levels.[7] Intensive activation of the RAAS and the sympathetic nervous system (SNS) is directly injurious to the heart and vasculature. These systems contribute to much of the LV remodeling that occurs during the progression of HF through myocyte hypertrophy, cellular proliferation, and development of fibrosis.[6] Of course, other mechanisms, including mechanical stressors (elevated filling pressures), cell dropout, oxidative stress, inflammation, and cytokine activity, also drive the remodeling process. Over time, augmented neurohormonal activity leads to further LV dysfunction and LV remodeling, including marked dilation and hypertrophy of the heart, essentially setting the stage for a vicious cycle.[3,8] This is the so-called neurohormonal hypothesis (**Fig. 1**).[8] The level of neurohormonal activation correlates strongly with the risk of HF progression and mortality.[9,10] ACE inhibitors, ARBs, aldosterone receptor blockers, and β-blockers have each been demonstrated to attenuate the remodeling process. The authors' thought is that the remodeling process is the hallmark of HF. The blockade of the adrenergic nervous system is seemingly critical toward prevention of the progression of the syndrome, and one can build a strong case based on animal and observational patient data that these drugs should be introduced as early therapy for patients who are stage B.[8,11,12]

ADVERSE EFFECTS OF NEUROHORMONAL SYSTEMS IN HF

The SNS evolved in mammalian species over a period of about 500 million years.[13] It presumably provided a survival advantage by allowing for an increase in cardiac output and improved flow to skeletal muscles at a time when cardiac output was impaired because of the reduced effective circulating volume. The RAAS and the SNS both evolved at about the same time as species moved from the saltwater ocean to land.[13,14] The evolution of the RAAS likely allowed for the species to survive despite the absence of ready access to salt and water. That is, these systems allowed the species to maintain blood pressure and perfusion to vital organs despite relative dehydration or volume loss. In addition to providing support for the fight-or-flight reaction, the SNS also provided protection against vascular collapse from excessive blood loss or volume depletion. Of course, the RAAS is an additionally powerful force in this respect. Although the SNS clearly plays a role in maintaining blood pressure to organs that are threatened by inadequate perfusion, the persistent activation of the SNS is likely harmful over time (**Box 1**).

The SNS increases heart rate and myocardial contractile force by stimulating the β1 receptors of the cardiac myocytes. This increased contractility comes at a price, especially if the myocardial oxygen equilibrium is threatened. Peripheral vasoconstriction raises the afterload and increases the impedance to the LV outflow. Increased afterload reduces cardiac systolic performance. Furthermore, persistent SNS activation indirectly stimulates several RAAS pathways that lead to increased myocardial collagen deposition and fibrosis. A classic experiment of nature is seen in patients with pheochromocytoma who develop either dilated or hypertrophic cardiomyopathy as a consequence of overly active SNS stimulation.[15] The SNS activation is associated with many cardiac rhythm disturbances, including lethal arrhythmias.

DIRECT CARDIOTOXIC EFFECTS OF NEUROHORMONES

Starling[16] recognized the potential detrimental effects of exogenous catecholamines in HF more than a century ago. Subsequently, Braunwald and colleagues[17–23] demonstrated the deleterious effects of the SNS in HF with a series of elegant

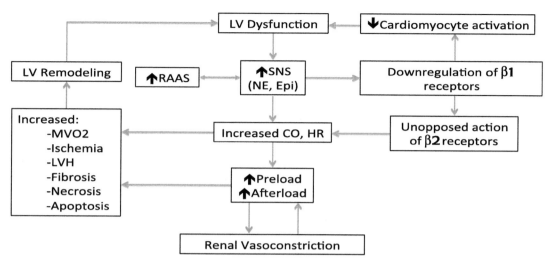

Fig. 1. The interaction of the sympathetic nervous system with cardiovascular system in HF. CO, cardiac output; Epi, epinephrine; HR, heart rate; LVH, LV hypertrophy; MVO2, myocardial oxygen consumption.

experiments in animals and humans. These experiments indicated that plasma norepinephrine concentration was often increased in patients with HF. They also observed a significant increase in 24-hour urinary norepinephrine excretion that correlated with the severity of HF. However, cardiac tissue norepinephrine concentration was remarkably low in patients with HF. This finding was recapitulated in animal models of HF. Furthermore, the responses of heart rate and of myocardial contraction to sympathetic stimulation in experimental HF were markedly impaired because of the downregulation of β-receptors and abnormal reflex control mechanisms.[17–23]

The mechanisms by which chronic activation of the adrenergic system leads to multiple deleterious effects on the cardiovascular system are complex. The β1-receptors downregulate in

response to excessive sympathetic drive (see **Fig. 1**).[24–28] This downregulation of β-receptors may serve as a compensatory protective mechanism against high concentrations of NE, which is directly toxic to cardiac myocytes.[29]

THE RATIONALE FOR β-ADRENERGIC BLOCKING THERAPY IN STAGE B, A PRECURSOR OF HF

As our understanding of the neurohormonal hypothesis advanced, the rationale for the use of β-blockers to treat patients with overt HF gradually became clearer. Although counterintuitive, early clinical experience using β-blocker in individual patients with HF was quite positive. Short-term treatment with β-blockers may reduce myocardial function, but experience with the long-term administration of β-blockers indicated a propensity to increase the EF and improve the clinical status of patients with HF.[12,30–36] β-blockers may reverse LV remodeling, reduce LV mass, and diminish LV volume. Lastly, β-blockers may benefit patients via the reduction in heart rate and by the diminishment of arrhythmias.[36] By the mid-1980s, there was increasing interest in the use of β-blockers for a treatment of HF, largely driven by the early Swedish experience in a few highly selected patients.[37–39]

We have learned from the Studies Of Left Ventricular Dysfunction-Prevention (SOLVD-Prevention)[40] that patients with asymptomatic LV dysfunction (stage B) are improved by ACE inhibitors.[40] There are now substantial data from patients who are stage B that β–blockers also prevent the progression of HF by reducing the LV

Box 1
Potential detrimental effects of the SNS on the cardiovascular system

Increased heart rate

Increased force of contraction

Increased blood pressure

Increased cell size of cardiac myocytes

Increased interstitial collagen deposition

Increased interstitial fibrosis

Direct toxic effect of catecholamines

Increased risk of arrhythmias

Increased potentiation of RAAS

chamber dimension and improving EF.[41,42] There are data indicating that metoprolol succinate is associated with reverse LV remodeling in patients who are stage B.[42] We know that neurohormones are progressively increased in patients with HF before the development of symptoms.[24] It follows that β-blockers should be introduced early (stage B) to prevent HF. However, there are no large clinical trials investigating β-blockers in a stage B cohort. Nevertheless, there has been broad consensus that β-blockers should be used in patients who are stage B. This strategy is also supported by current guidelines.[1] Numerous small observational studies have rather consistently indicated that various β-blockers, including carvedilol, metoprolol succinate, and metoprolol tartrate, as well as non–β-blocker bradycardic ionophores, such as ivabradine, can reduce the LV chamber size and improve systolic performance. When β-blockers are used in patients with stage CHF, there is seemingly a consistent improvement in LVEF, averaging about 7 EF units per patient, with a reduction in end-diastolic volume, similar to what is found with ACE inhibitors and ARBs.

CLINICAL TRIALS OF β-ADRENERGIC BLOCKERS IN PATIENTS WITH HF

The distinguishing characteristic of stage B is asymptomatic LV dysfunction. Stage B includes patients with either underlying structural heart disease, such as LV hypertrophy (LVH), or functional abnormalities, such as a low LVEF. The authors recognize that there are no large, randomized clinical trials specifically addressing the use of β-blockers in patients who are stage B. Virtually all large randomized controlled trials (RCTs) have been performed in patients with New York Heart Association (NYHA) class II to IV (stage C and D). We here in review the landmark RCTs leading to the approval of β-blockers for the treatment of HF and subsequently examine what data they have in patients with stage B treated with β-blockers.

β-Adrenergic Blockers for Stage C and D

Because conventional wisdom dictated that HF was caused by a decline in systolic function, for many years it was thought that β-blockers were contraindicated.[43,44] In fact, initial small studies demonstrated negative inotropic effects and a poor clinical response to β-blockers, reemphasizing this view. Consequently, early clinical trials of β-blockers in hypertension and in patients with acute myocardial infarction excluded patients with HF.

Waagstein and colleagues[37] were the first to demonstrate that lowering the heart rate with a β-blocker provided benefit to patients with HF. This achievement occurred when Waagstein and colleagues[37] administered practolol to a single patient with HF who demonstrated dramatic clinical improvement. Subsequently, this group went on to demonstrate that β-blockers improved patients with HF in a series of case reports.[38,39,45] Thereafter, the metoprolol in dilated cardiomyopathy (MDC) was designed by the group from Gothenburg, Sweden and Bristow's[46] group from University of Utah. These collaborators assessed the impact of metoprolol on the primary end point of death or progression to heart transplantation. This trial, although largely underpowered, was the first randomized controlled clinical trial to examine the use of β-blockers (metoprolol tartrate) in patients with HF. A total of 383 patients were randomized, 10 of which were asymptomatic. All had an LVEF less than 40%. The trial indicated a nonsignificant trend in favor of metoprolol but this was largely driven by a reduction in a perceived need for heart transplantation, a rather subjective end point.[46] Nevertheless, this study was a turning point in the development of future trials using β-blockers to treat HF.

The Metoprolol CR/XL Randomized Intervention Trial in Chronic Heart Failure (MERIT-HF), randomized 3991 patients with symptomatic HF and LVEF less than 40% to controlled-release metoprolol versus placebo. After a 12-month follow-up, metoprolol succinate reduced all-cause mortality risk by 34% ($P = .006$) and total mortality or all-cause hospitalization risk by 19% ($P<.001$) (**Fig. 2**). The risk of sudden death was reduced by 41% ($P<.001$) and risk of death caused by worsening HF by 49% ($P = .002$). Compared with placebo, metoprolol succinate reduced the total length of hospitalization from all causes by 17% and 36% for hospitalization caused by HF.[47] It should be noted that patients randomized in the United States to the MERIT-HF trial derived no survival benefit.

The Cardiac Insufficiency Bisoprolol Study II (CIBIS II) compared the effects of bisoprolol, a selective β1-antagonist, with placebo in 2647 symptomatic patients (NYHA class III or IV) and LVEF less than or equal to 35% receiving standard therapy (ACE inhibitors and diuretics).[30] During a mean follow-up of 1.3 years, bisoprolol significantly reduced the primary end point of all-cause mortality by 34% (17% vs 12%, $P<.0001$) (**Fig. 3**). Bisoprolol also resulted in significantly fewer cardiac deaths ($P = .0049$) and hospitalization for any cause ($P = .0006$) or for worsening HF (32% reduction compared with placebo;

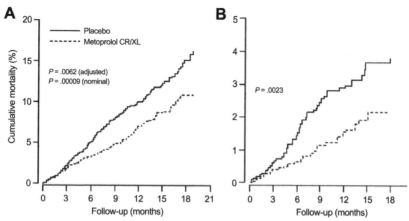

Fig. 2. The effect of metoprolol CR/XL versus placebo on mortality (*A*) and worsening HF (*B*). (*From* Effect of metoprolol CR/XL in chronic heart failure: metoprolol CR/XL randomised intervention trial in congestive heart failure (MERIT-HF). Lancet 1999;353(9169):2001–7; with permission.)

P<.0001). In an open-label study of 201 patients, mean LVEF improved after 3 months of therapy (31% at baseline and 41% after bisoprolol; *P*<.0001). Bisoprolol significantly decreased end-systolic and end-diastolic LV diameters (4.9 mm and 2.3 mm, respectively; *P*<.0001 for both remodeling indices).[30,48] Bisoprolol is largely used in Europe, and there is little experience using it in the United States for the treatment of HF.

The Beta-Blocker Evaluation of Survival Trial (BEST) studied the effects of bucindolol, a nonselective β-adrenergic antagonist, which indicated a nonsignificant reduction in all-cause mortality (*P* = .13).[49] The reasons why the study failed to meet its end point are still widely debated. The less than robust outcome may have been because of a genetic polymorphism involving the β1 receptor gene, which may have impacted the response to bucindolol.

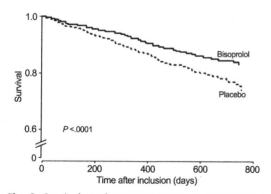

Fig. 3. Survival Kaplan-Meier curves in CIBIS-II trial. This graph shows the evidence of early separation of the curves within the first 6 months.

Carvedilol was tested in the US Carvedilol Heart Failure Program in a series of clinical trials involving mild to severe HF.[50] Each individual study had a run-in period. The total program included 1094 patients with chronic HF that were randomized to one of the 4 arms of the study on the basis of their exercise capacity. Within each of the different trial protocols, patients with mild, moderate, or severe HF and LVEF less than 35% were randomized to carvedilol (n = 696) or placebo (n = 398) with the combined end point of death or hospitalization. Carvedilol therapy was associated with a significant 65% reduction in overall mortality rate (3.2% vs 7.8%; *P*<.001). Carvedilol therapy also resulted in a reduction of the hospitalizations for cardiovascular causes by 27% (*P* = .04) and a 38% reduction in the combined end point of hospitalization or death (*P*<.001).[50] In one of the studies from the US Carvedilol Heart Failure Program that included 366 patients with mild HF (NYHA class II) who were randomized to either carvedilol (6.25–50.0 mg twice daily) or placebo, carvedilol-treated patients had a statistically significant LVEF improvement compared with patients receiving placebo (10% vs 3%, respectively; *P*<.001) at the 12-month follow-up.[12]

A similar beneficial effect of reduction in mortality and hospitalization was observed in the Australia/New Zealand Heart Failure Research Collaborative Group (ANZ) trial.[51] In this study, 415 patients with chronic, stable HF were randomly assigned to carvedilol or placebo and followed up for an average of 19 months. Carvedilol resulted in a 26% reduction in the risk of all-cause mortality or hospitalization (95% confidence interval [CI], 0.57–0.95) compared with placebo. End-diastolic and end-systolic dimensions decreased by 3.2 mm ($P = .06$) and 1.7 mm ($P = .001$), respectively, resulting in a 5.3% ($P<.0001$) increase in LVEF in carvedilol-treated patients.[51]

The effectiveness of β-blockers in slowing the progression of HF is well demonstrated in NYHA classes II to IV. In these trials, there were few asymptomatic patients. There were 2.5% asymptomatic patients in the MDC trial, 0.5% in the MERIT trial, and 30% in ANZ trial. The BEST and CIBIS-II trials did not include any patients with stage B.

β-Adrenergic Blockers and Stage B

In the SOLVD-Prevention trial, 24% of patients were on treatment with β-blockers.[40] A post hoc analysis of the SOLVD-Prevention trial demonstrates that patients on β-blockers who were asymptomatic had a significant reduction of death and development of HF.[52] This retrospective analysis suggests that β-blockers reduce mortality and pump failure in a cohort of patients who were essentially stage B. In addition, the adjusted survival analysis indicates that trial participants receiving both β-blocker and enalapril had an independent reduction in the risk of death, mainly arrhythmic and cardiac failure death, and a slower progression to symptomatic HF as assessed by the composite end point of death and hospitalization for HF. Although a post hoc analysis, the study by Exner and colleagues[52] supports the use of β-blockers in patients who are stage B to prevent HF from developing to a more advanced and lethal entity.

The REversal of VEntricular Remodeling with Toprol-XL (REVERT) trial was a study of patients with LVEF less than 40%, mild LV dilation, and no symptoms of HF (NYHA class I).[42] The results of this small study indicated that β-blocker therapy can reduce remodeling in patients who are stage B.

ROLE OF BRADYCARDIA IN THE TREATMENT OF HEART FAILURE

An increased resting heart rate is associated with higher total and cardiovascular mortality.[53] Patients with HF and a heart rate more than 70 beats per minute have a significantly greater cardiovascular mortality and risk for hospital admission than those with a heart rate less than 70 beats per minute. The discrimination by heart rate is better for HF than for coronary vascular outcomes.[54,55] Several recent trials in patients with HF suggest an association of reduction in mortality with the magnitude of heart rate reduction.[53] Thus, one of the fundamental questions is whether or not it is mainly the lower heart rate that leads to marked benefit of β-blockers in the treatment of patients with HF. Could there be some other important contribution, such as reduced contractility? The benefit of β-blockers therapy is substantially mitigated when the heart is paced at a faster heart rate in animal studies, suggesting that a slower heart rate is most beneficial in HF. The idea that just slowing the heart rate may be a fundamental benefit for patients with HF remains intriguing.

With this background, some investigators have focused on an ionophore molecule that can reduce the heart rate without interaction on LV performance. Ivabradine, a new bradycardia-inducing agent with no negative inotropic properties, acts on the I_f-channel. The f in I_f stands for *funny* because this ion channel has funny/unusual properties. This channel is activated by hyperpolarization and is regulated not by phosphorylation through protein kinase A in response to increased intracellular cyclic adenosine monophosphate (cAMP), but by direct binding of cAMP. cAMP is the second messenger molecule that integrates intracellularly the balance between cardiac sympathetic nerves. Sympathetic nerves increase cAMP through the action of norepinephrine on surface β1- and β2-adrenoceptors and subsequent activation of the G-protein Gs. Cardiac vagal nerves decrease cAMP through the action of acetylcholine on surface muscarinic receptors and through subsequent activation of the inhibitory G-protein Gi.[56]

It has been suggested that ivabradine may improve LV function in animal models via a simple reduction in heart rate.[56–58] Ivabradine benefited patients with coronary artery disease and LV dysfunction in the BEAUTIFUL trial (Morbidity-Mortality Evaluation of the I_f Inhibitor Ivabradine in Patients With Coronary Artery Disease and Left Ventricular Dysfunction). These benefits were largely a reduction in coronary events.[55] The SHIFT study (Systolic Heart Failure Treatment with the I_f Inhibitor Ivabradine Trial) by Swedberg and colleagues[59] assigned 6558 patients with HF to ivabradine (n = 3268) or placebo (n = 3290). Entry was restricted to patient with symptomatic HF with LVEF less than 35% and sinus rhythm with a resting heart rate of more than 70 beats per minute. The primary end point of the study was a composite of cardiovascular death or hospitalization for worsening HF. During a median follow-up of 23 months, 24% of the patients in the ivabradine group and 29% of those taking placebo had a primary end point event (hazard ratio [HR] 0.82; 95% CI 0.75–0.90; $P<.0001$) (**Fig. 4**). The effects were driven mainly by reduced hospital admissions for worsening HF (21%

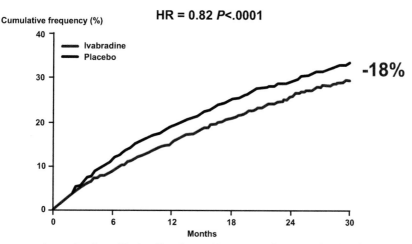

HR = 0.82 P<.0001

-18%

Fig. 4. Primary composite end point of ivabradine (n = 793; 14.5% PY) versus placebo. (n = 937; 17.7% PY).

placebo vs 16% ivabradine; HR 0.74; 0.66–0.83; P<.0001) and deaths caused by HF (5% vs 3%; HR 0.74; 0.58–0.94; P = .014). Fewer serious adverse events occurred in the ivabradine group (3388 events) than in the placebo group (3847; P = .025). The patients assigned to ivabradine had a 5 times higher risk of symptomatic bradycardia compared with the placebo group (P<.0001). Visual side effects were reported by 3% of the patients on ivabradine and 17 (1%) on placebo (P<.0001).[59]

The benefit of ivabradine in the SHIFT study was related to the magnitude of the heart rate reduction. Ivabradine also attenuates adverse remodeling and improves angiogenesis after myocardial infarction in rats. This finding suggests that heart rate reduction alone may have a powerful antiremodeling effect.[56,57,60] However, a critical question still to be answered is whether the heart rate slowing effect or negative inotropic effect is more important in providing benefit from β-adrenergic–blocking drugs.

SUMMARY

β-Blockers are an important treatment of HF and have proved useful in reducing the progression of the syndrome. They should be considered for patients with asymptomatic LV dysfunction. Evidence-based β-blocker therapy (bisoprolol, carvedilol, or metoprolol succinate) in combination with standard therapy is a mainstay for the treatment of all symptomatic patients with LV systolic dysfunction. Patients in stage B very likely also benefit from the early introduction of β-blockers, but there are no large randomized clinical trials to support this strategy. Whether there is a role of for ivabradine in the treatment of HF is still not clear. So far, there is only one large RCT available.

This class of medications has not been tested in patients who are stage B.

REFERENCES

1. Hunt SA, Abraham WT, Chin MH, et al. 2009 focused update incorporated into the ACC/AHA 2005 guidelines for the diagnosis and management of heart failure in adults A report of the American College of Cardiology Foundation/American Heart Association task force on practice guidelines developed in collaboration with the international society for heart and lung transplantation. J Am Coll Cardiol 2009; 53(15):e1–90.
2. Bristow MR. Treatment of chronic heart failure with beta-adrenergic receptor antagonists: a convergence of receptor pharmacology and clinical cardiology. Circ Res 2011;109(10):1176–94.
3. Cohn JN, Ferrari R, Sharpe N. Cardiac remodeling–concepts and clinical implications: a consensus paper from an international forum on cardiac remodeling. Behalf of an international forum on cardiac remodeling. J Am Coll Cardiol 2000;35(3): 569–82.
4. Vaughan DE, Pfeffer MA. Angiotensin converting enzyme inhibitors and cardiovascular remodelling. Cardiovasc Res 1994;28(2):159–65.
5. van Campen LC, Visser FC, Visser CA. Ejection fraction improvement by beta-blocker treatment in patients with heart failure: an analysis of studies published in the literature. J Cardiovasc Pharmacol 1998;32(Suppl 1):S31–5.
6. Mann DL, Bristow MR. Mechanisms and models in heart failure: the biomechanical model and beyond. Circulation 2005;111(21):2837–49.
7. Schrier RW, Abraham WT. Hormones and hemodynamics in heart failure. N Engl J Med 1999;341(8): 577–85.

8. Packer M. The neurohormonal hypothesis: a theory to explain the mechanism of disease progression in heart failure. J Am Coll Cardiol 1992;20(1):248–54.

9. Cohn JN, Levine TB, Olivari MT, et al. Plasma norepinephrine as a guide to prognosis in patients with chronic congestive heart failure. N Engl J Med 1984;311(13):819–23.

10. Francis GS, Cohn JN, Johnson G, et al. Plasma norepinephrine, plasma renin activity, and congestive heart failure. Relations to survival and the effects of therapy in V-HeFT II. The V-HeFT VA cooperative studies group. Circulation 1993;87(Suppl 6):VI40–8.

11. Vantrimpont P, Rouleau JL, Wun CC, et al. Additive beneficial effects of beta-blockers to angiotensin-converting enzyme inhibitors in the survival and ventricular enlargement (SAVE) study. SAVE investigators. J Am Coll Cardiol 1997;29(2):229–36.

12. Colucci WS, Packer M, Bristow MR, et al. Carvedilol inhibits clinical progression in patients with mild symptoms of heart failure. US carvedilol heart failure study group. Circulation 1996;94(11):2800–6.

13. Harris P. Evolution and the cardiac patient. Cardiovasc Res 1983;17(8):437–45.

14. Harris P. Evolution and the cardiac patient. Cardiovasc Res 1983;17(6):313–9.

15. Gatzoulis KA, Tolis G, Theopistou A, et al. Cardiomyopathy due to a pheochromocytoma. A reversible entity. Acta Cardiol 1998;53(4):227–9.

16. Starling EH. The linacre lecture on the law of the heart. London (UK): Longmans, Green and Co; 1918.

17. Chidsey CA, Braunwald E. Sympathetic activity and neurotransmitter depletion in congestive heart failure. Pharmacol Rev 1966;18(1):685–700.

18. Chidsey CA, Sonnenblick EH, Morrow AG, et al. Norepinephrine stores and contractile force of papillary muscle from the failing human heart. Circulation 1966;33(1):43–51.

19. Chidsey CA, Braunwald E, Morrow AG. Catecholamine excretion and cardiac stores of norepinephrine in congestive heart failure. Am J Med 1965;39:442–51.

20. Chidsey CA, Kaiser GA, Sonnenblick EH, et al. Cardiac norepinephrine stores in experimental heart failure in the dog. J Clin Invest 1964;43:2386–93.

21. Chidsey CA, Braunwald E, Morrow AG, et al. Myocardial norepinephrine concentration in man. Effects of reserpine and of congestive heart failure. N Engl J Med 1963;269:653–8.

22. Chidsey CA, Harrison DC, Braunwald E. Augmentation of the plasma nor-epinephrine response to exercise in patients with congestive heart failure. N Engl J Med 1962;267:650–4.

23. Braunwald E, Chidsey CA. The adrenergic nervous system in the control of the normal and failing heart. Proc R Soc Med 1965;58(12):1063–6.

24. Francis GS, Benedict C, Johnstone DE, et al. Comparison of neuroendocrine activation in patients with left ventricular dysfunction with and without congestive heart failure. A substudy of the studies of left ventricular dysfunction (SOLVD). Circulation 1990;82(5):1724–9.

25. Levine TB, Francis GS, Goldsmith SR, et al. Activity of the sympathetic nervous system and renin-angiotensin system assessed by plasma hormone levels and their relation to hemodynamic abnormalities in congestive heart failure. Am J Cardiol 1982;49(7):1659–66.

26. Mann DL, Cooper G 4th. Neurohumoral activation in congestive heart failure: a double-edged sword? Clin Cardiol 1989;12(9):485–90.

27. Foody JM, Farrell MH, Krumholz HM. Beta-blocker therapy in heart failure: scientific review. JAMA 2002;287(7):883–9.

28. Bristow MR. Mechanism of action of beta-blocking agents in heart failure. Am J Cardiol 1997;80(11A):26L–40L.

29. Mann DL, Kent RL, Parsons B, et al. Adrenergic effects on the biology of the adult mammalian cardiocyte. Circulation 1992;85(2):790–804.

30. Anthonio RL, Brouwer J, Lechat P, et al. Different effects of bisoprolol on heart rate in patients with ischemic or idiopathic dilated cardiomyopathy (a 24-hour Holter substudy of the Cardiac Insufficiency Bisoprolol Study [CIBIS]). Am J Cardiol 1999;83(8):1286–9, A10.

31. Cohn JN, Johnson GR, Shabetai R, et al. Ejection fraction, peak exercise oxygen consumption, cardiothoracic ratio, ventricular arrhythmias, and plasma norepinephrine as determinants of prognosis in heart failure. The V-HeFT VA cooperative studies group. Circulation 1993;87(Suppl 6):VI5–16.

32. Gilbert EM, Abraham WT, Olsen S, et al. Comparative hemodynamic, left ventricular functional, and antiadrenergic effects of chronic treatment with metoprolol versus carvedilol in the failing heart. Circulation 1996;94(11):2817–25.

33. Bristow MR, O'Connell JB, Gilbert EM, et al. Dose-response of chronic beta-blocker treatment in heart failure from either idiopathic dilated or ischemic cardiomyopathy. Bucindolol investigators. Circulation 1994;89(4):1632–42.

34. Eichhorn EJ. The paradox of beta-adrenergic blockade for the management of congestive heart failure. Am J Med 1992;92(5):527–38.

35. Bristow MR, Gilbert EM, Abraham WT, et al. Carvedilol produces dose-related improvements in left ventricular function and survival in subjects with chronic heart failure. MOCHA investigators. Circulation 1996;94(11):2807–16.

36. Lechat P, Hulot JS, Escolano S, et al. Heart rate and cardiac rhythm relationships with bisoprolol benefit in chronic heart failure in CIBIS II trial. Circulation 2001;103(10):1428–33.

37. Waagstein F, Hjalmarson A, Varnauskas E, et al. Effect of chronic beta-adrenergic receptor blockade

in congestive cardiomyopathy. Br Heart J 1975; 37(10):1022–36.

38. Waagstein F, Hjalmarson AC. Effect of cardioselective beta-blockade on heart function and chest pain in acute myocardial infarction. Acta Med Scand Suppl 1976;587:193–200.

39. Waagstein F, Hjalmarson AC. Double-blind study of the effect of cardioselective beta-blockade on chest pain in acute myocardial infarction. Acta Med Scand Suppl 1976;587:201–8.

40. Effect of enalapril on mortality and the development of heart failure in asymptomatic patients with reduced left ventricular ejection fractions. The SOLVD investigators. N Engl J Med 1992;327(10):685–91.

41. Sharpe N, Doughty RN. Left ventricular remodelling and improved long-term outcomes in chronic heart failure. Eur Heart J 1998;19(Suppl B):B36–9.

42. Colucci WS, Kolias TJ, Adams KF, et al. Metoprolol reverses left ventricular remodeling in patients with asymptomatic systolic dysfunction: the REversal of VEntricular Remodeling with Toprol-XL (REVERT) trial. Circulation 2007;116(1):49–56.

43. Currie PJ, Kelly MJ, McKenzie A, et al. Oral beta-adrenergic blockade with metoprolol in chronic severe dilated cardiomyopathy. J Am Coll Cardiol 1984;3(1):203–9.

44. Ikram H, Fitzpatrick D. Double-blind trial of chronic oral beta blockade in congestive cardiomyopathy. Lancet 1981;2(8245):490–3.

45. Waagstein F, Reiz S, Ariniego R, et al. Clinical results with prenalterol in patients with heart failure. Am Heart J 1981;102(3 Pt 2):548–54.

46. Waagstein F, Bristow MR, Swedberg K, et al. Beneficial effects of metoprolol in idiopathic dilated cardiomyopathy. Metoprolol in dilated cardiomyopathy (MDC) trial study group. Lancet 1993;342(8885):1441–6.

47. Merit Investigator. Effect of metoprolol CR/XL in chronic heart failure: metoprolol CR/XL randomised intervention trial in congestive heart failure (MERIT-HF). Lancet 1999;353(9169):2001–7.

48. de Groote P, Delour P, Lamblin N, et al. Effects of bisoprolol in patients with stable congestive heart failure. Ann Cardiol Angeiol (Paris) 2004;53(4):167–70.

49. Domanski MJ, Krause-Steinrauf H, Massie BM, et al. A comparative analysis of the results from 4 trials of beta-blocker therapy for heart failure: BEST, CIBIS-II, MERIT-HF, and COPERNICUS. J Card Fail 2003; 9(5):354–63.

50. Packer M, Bristow MR, Cohn JN, et al. The effect of carvedilol on morbidity and mortality in patients with chronic heart failure. U.S. carvedilol heart failure study group. N Engl J Med 1996;334(21):1349–55.

51. Australia/New Zealand Heart Failure Research Collaborative Group. Randomised, placebo-controlled trial of carvedilol in patients with congestive heart failure due to ischaemic heart disease. Australia/New Zealand heart failure research collaborative group. Lancet 1997;349(9049):375–80.

52. Exner DV, Dries DL, Waclawiw MA, et al. Beta-adrenergic blocking agent use and mortality in patients with asymptomatic and symptomatic left ventricular systolic dysfunction: a post hoc analysis of the studies of left ventricular dysfunction. J Am Coll Cardiol 1999;33(4):916–23.

53. Fox K, Borer JS, Camm AJ, et al. Resting heart rate in cardiovascular disease. J Am Coll Cardiol 2007; 50(9):823–30.

54. Fox K, Ford I, Steg PG, et al. BEAUTIFUL investigators. Heart rate as a prognostic risk factor in patients with coronary artery disease and left-ventricular systolic dysfunction (BEAUTIFUL): a subgroup analysis of a randomised controlled trial. Lancet 2008; 372(9641):817–21.

55. Fox K, Ford I, Steg PG, et al. BEAUTIFUL investigators. Ivabradine for patients with stable coronary artery disease and left-ventricular systolic dysfunction (BEAUTIFUL): a randomised, double-blind, placebo-controlled trial. Lancet 2008;372(9641): 807–16.

56. Heusch G, Skyschally A, Gres P, et al. Improvement of regional myocardial blood flow and function and reduction of infarct size with ivabradine: protection beyond heart rate reduction. Eur Heart J 2008; 29(18):2265–75.

57. Heusch G. Heart rate in the pathophysiology of coronary blood flow and myocardial ischaemia: benefit from selective bradycardic agents. Br J Pharmacol 2008;153(8):1589–601.

58. Sata Y, Krum H. The future of pharmacological therapy for heart failure. Circ J 2010;74(5):809–17.

59. Swedberg K, Komajda M, Bohm M, et al, SHIFT Investigators. Ivabradine and outcomes in chronic heart failure (SHIFT): a randomised placebo-controlled study. Lancet 2010;376(9744):875–85.

60. Bohm M, Swedberg K, Komajda M, et al, SHIFT Investigators. Heart rate as a risk factor in chronic heart failure (SHIFT): the association between heart rate and outcomes in a randomised placebo-controlled trial. Lancet 2010;376(9744): 886–94.

The Role of Mineralocorticoid Receptor Antagonists in Patients with American College of Cardiology/American Heart Association Stage B Heart Failure

Bertram Pitt, MD

KEYWORDS
- ACC/AHA • Heart failure • Mineralocorticoid
- Left ventricular hypertrophy

An increase in plasma aldosterone and cortisol levels, both of which can activate the mineralocorticoid receptor (MR), has been shown to be associated with an increased risk of cardiovascular mortality and hospitalizations for heart failure (HF) in patients with chronic HF.[1] MR antagonists (MRAs) have been shown to be effective in reducing total mortality as well as hospitalizations for HF in patients with chronic HF, a reduced left ventricular ejection fraction, as well as HF and reduced left ventricular ejection fraction (HFREF) early after myocardial infarction (MI).[2–4] Mineralocorticoid antagonists have also been shown to improve diastolic function in patients with HF and a preserved left ventricular ejection fraction (HFPEF),[5] and the MRA spironolactone is currently being studied in the National Heart, Lung, and Blood Institute TOPCAT (Treatment of Preserved Cardiac Function Heart Failure with an Aldosterone Antagonist) trial.[6] Increased plasma aldosterone levels have also been associated with an increase in cardiovascular events in patients with MI independent of the presence of HF,[7] and

MRAs are currently under investigation in patients early after MI without clinical evidence or a history of HF.[8] The role of MRAs on cardiovascular outcomes in patients with American College of Cardiology/American Heart Association (ACC/AHA) stage B HF has not, however, as yet been evaluated in large-scale prospective randomized trials. There is, however, increasing evidence to suggest that MRAs will play an important role in preventing the development of HF in patients with ACC/AHA stage B HF in the future.

RATIONALE FOR THE USE OF MRAs IN PATIENTS WITH STAGE B HF

Stage B HF as defined by the ACC/AHA guidelines[9] includes patients who have developed structural heart disease that is strongly associated with the development of HF but who have never had signs or symptoms of HF. The structural abnormalities associated with the development of HF include left ventricular hypertrophy (LVH) and fibrosis, often caused by hypertension,

Cardiovascular Center, University Hospital, University of Michigan School of Medicine, 1500 East Medical Center Drive, SPC 5853, Suite 2722K, Ann Arbor, MI 48109-5853, USA
E-mail address: bpitt@umich.edu

Heart Failure Clin 8 (2012) 247–253
doi:10.1016/j.hfc.2011.11.001
1551-7136/12/$ – see front matter © 2012 Published by Elsevier Inc

diabetes mellitus, and/or visceral obesity with the metabolic syndrome. Stage B HF also includes patients with asymptomatic left ventricular dilatation due to nonischemic or ischemic cardiomyopathy, those with asymptomatic valvular heart disease, and those with a prior MI without evidence of HF. This article focuses on the potential role of MRAs in patients with stage B HF due to hypertension, diabetes mellitus, and/or visceral obesity with the metabolic syndrome and briefly discusses the role of MRAs in patients with left ventricular dilatation due to nonischemic or ischemic cardiomyopathy and in those with a prior MI but without left ventricular dilatation or evidence of HF.

MRAs IN PATIENTS WITH HYPERTENSIVE HEART DISEASE

Lowering of blood pressure in patients with essential hypertension has been shown to be effective in preventing the development and progression of LVH. Although all classes of antihypertensive medications seem to be effective in preventing LVH, there is reason to believe that in certain circumstances MRAs may be particularly effective and that they may have important blood pressure–independent effects.

For example, in patients with resistant hypertension (ie, those patients whose blood pressure cannot be controlled by 3 or more antihypertensive agents at effective doses, including a diuretic, angiotensin-converting enzyme inhibitor [ACE-I] or angiotensin receptor blocking agent [ARB], and a calcium channel blocking agent [CCB]) who are at increased risk of developing LVH and HF, studies have shown that relatively small doses of an MRA such as spironolactone, 12.5 to 25 mg/d, can markedly reduce blood pressure independent of the renin-aldosterone ratio.[10] One clue to the potential effects of MRAs independent of their effect on lowering blood pressure comes from a comparison of patients with primary aldosteronism with those with essential hypertension at a similar blood pressure.[11,12] Patients with primary aldosteronism have a significant increase in the incidence of LVH and HF as well as an increase in MI, stroke, atrial fibrillation, urinary albuminuria, the metabolic syndrome, and sudden cardiac death. A blood pressure–independent effect of MRAs is also suggested by a study in patients with stage 1 hypertension in which the β-adrenergic blocking agent atenolol was compared with the MRA eplerenone.[13] Patients randomized to atenolol had a significant increase in vascular stiffness and resistance compared with those randomized

to eplerenone who had a decrease in vascular stiffness, a decreased ratio of collagen/elastin, and a reduction in inflammatory cytokines independent of a reduction in blood pressure. In a study comparing the effects of the dihydropyridine calcium channel blocking agent amlodipine with the ARB losartan in patients with hypertensive heart disease and LVH, plasma aldosterone levels were a blood pressure–independent predictor of left ventricular mass regression and the patients who had both a reduction in plasma aldosterone levels and blood pressure had the best reduction in left ventricular mass.[14] Plasma aldosterone levels have been shown to correlate with left ventricular mass and vascular stiffness,[15,16] whereas MRAs reduce both left ventricular mass and vascular stiffness. MRAs have also been shown to be important in preventing the development of myocardial fibrosis in both animal models and in patients with hypertensive heart disease as well as in those after MI.[17,18] Myocardial fibrosis due to hypertension, visceral obesity, and/or diabetes mellitus often precedes the development of LVH.[19] Increasing evidence suggests that myocardial fibrosis plays an important role in the transition from hypertensive and diabetic heart disease to diastolic HF or HFPEF. Myocardial fibrosis has also been implicated in the development of ventricular arrhythmias and sudden cardiac death in patients with hypertensive heart disease, with diabetes mellitus, and after MI. Myocardial fibrosis causes an inhomogeneity of electrical conduction and impairs gap junction function.[20,21] MRAs prevent nuclear factor κβ and AP-1 signaling, inflammatory cytokine activation, vascular inflammation, and subsequent myocardial fibrosis.[22,23] An aldosterone-induced increase in osteopontin may be particularly important in the development of myocardial fibrosis because in osteopontin knockout mice, the effects of aldosterone on myocardial fibrosis are significantly reduced.[24] Recently, the role of the macrophage has been shown to be of importance in aldosterone and MR-induced myocardial fibrosis and hypertrophy. Macrophages have been shown to express MRs, and knockout of the macrophage MR has been shown to prevent aldosterone-induced myocardial fibrosis and hypertrophy.[25]

A further clue to the potential role of MRAs in preventing the development of manifest HF in patients with stage B HF comes from experimental studies of aortic banding with the subsequent development of LVH.[26] In this study, the development of LVH resulted in an upregulation of the brain RAAS with subsequent central sympathetic nervous system and inflammatory cytokine activation, which could be blocked by an MRA. Blockade of central sympathetic activation in patients with LVH would have important implications for preventing not only the development of HF but also the occurrence of sudden cardiac death, a major risk in patients with hypertensive heart disease and LVH.

In the 4E (Eplerenone, Enalapril and Eplerenone/Enalapril Combination Therapy in Patients with Left Ventricular Hypertrophy) trial[27] of patients with hypertensive heart disease and LVH detected by echocardiography, patients underwent magnetic resonance imaging (MRI) analysis of left ventricular mass and were then randomized to the ACE-I enalapril, the MRA eplerenone, or their combination and were followed up for 9 months along with repeated determination of left ventricular mass by MRI. Both enalapril and eplerenone were effective in reducing left ventricular mass and urinary albuminuria. However, the combination of ACE-I and MRA seemed to be more effective than eplerenone alone. Of interest was the finding that the reduction in left ventricular mass and urinary albuminuria by the combination of enalapril and eplerenone seemed to be independent of the reduction in blood pressure and occurred with normal plasma aldosterone levels. The reduction in left ventricular mass by eplerenone in patients with a normal plasma aldosterone level can be explained by the fact that the MR can be activated by cortisol as well as aldosterone. Cortisol has a greater affinity for MR than aldosterone, but, in renal tubular epithelial cells, the enzyme 11β-HSD2 that converts cortisol to cortisone, which cannot activate the MR, is abundant such that under normal circumstances cortisol is not available to activate the MR.[28] However, in essential hypertension, this enzyme may be downregulated such that cortisol can activate the MR.[29] This enzyme is less abundant or absent in the myocardium such that cortisol occupies but normally does not activate the MR. However, under conditions of increased oxidative stress, cortisol may activate the MR. MRAs such as spironolactone and eplerenone block the genomic activation of the MR either by aldosterone or by cortisol.[29]

ROLE OF MRAs ON IMPORTANT COMORBID CONDITIONS TRIGGERING THE DEVELOPMENT OF MANIFEST HF IN STAGE B

One factor suggesting an important role of MRAs in preventing the development of manifest HF in patients with stage B HF is the finding that patients with hypertensive heart disease and visceral obesity with myocardial fibrosis and/or LVH often have concomitant sleep apnea. Recurrent episodes of hypoxia during sleep apnea are associated with inflammatory cytokine activation and a decrease in endothelial nitric oxide availability

with subsequent hypertension and its associated target organ damage. Aldosterone levels have been found to be elevated in patients with sleep apnea and to correlate with the number of hypoxic episodes[30] and are thought to play an important role in the progression of hypertensive heart disease associated with sleep apnea. Similarly, aldosterone levels are elevated in patients with atrial fibrillation.[31] Recently, MRAs have been shown to prevent the development of atrial fibrillation in patients with HFREF (Swedberg K, Zannad F, McMurray J, et al. Eplerenone and atrial fibrillation in mild systolic heart failure—results from the eplerenone in mild patients hospitalization and survival study in heart failure [EMPHASIS-HF] study. Submitted for publication, 2011). Aldosterone by causing left atrial fibrosis, remodeling, and decreasing nitric oxide availability in the atria predisposes to the development of atrial fibrillation, which is an important trigger for the development of manifest HF in patients in stage B.

Aldosterone has also been shown to be associated with pancreatic beta-cell dysfunction, and aldosterone levels have been found to be elevated in patients with visceral obesity and the metabolic syndrome.[32,33] The adipocyte releases substances such as rac-1, which can stimulate adrenal production of aldosterone.[34] Thus, MRAs may have an important role in preventing the progression of myocardial fibrosis, LVH, and the development of HFPEF in patients with the metabolic syndrome.

Patients with hypertensive heart disease, visceral obesity, and/or diabetes mellitus with left ventricular fibrosis and/or hypertrophy often have concomitant coronary artery disease. Myocardial ischemia with resultant diastolic and/or systolic dysfunction is another important trigger for the precipitation of manifest HF in patients with stage B HF. Recent data from the LURIC (Ludwigshafen Risk and Cardiovascular Health) study[7] suggest that plasma aldosterone levels in patients with coronary artery disease independent of the presence of MI, HF, or hypertension predict the development of cardiovascular events, including HF. There is increasing evidence linking activation of the MR to the development and progression of atherosclerosis and its clinical consequences: MI, stroke, and sudden cardiac death.[35] Aldosterone causes a reduction in the enzyme glucose 6 phosphate dehydrogenase[36] with a resultant decrease in glutathione levels and antioxidant reserves and a resultant increase in reactive oxygen species and decrease in nitric oxide availability. MRAs alone and in conjunction with an ACE-I have been shown to improve endothelial dysfunction, an important prognostic indicator in patients with HF, and to impede the progression of experimental atherosclerosis in a lipid-fed rabbit model,[37] the apolipoprotein E knockout mouse,[38] and nonhuman primates.[39] Thus, MRAs may play an important role in preventing myocardial ischemia, an important trigger of manifest HF, in patients in stage B HF with myocardial fibrosis and/or LVH due to hypertensive heart disease and/or diabetes mellitus and concomitant coronary artery disease. MRAs may also play an important role in patients with MI but without clinical evidence of HF by preventing reactive fibrosis in noninfarcted areas of the left ventricle and ventricular remodeling.[40]

THE ROLE OF ACE-I AND/OR ARB IN PREVENTING THE PRODUCTION OF ALDOSTERONE FROM THE ADRENAL GLAND

Activation of the angiotensin type 1 receptor (AT1-R) is an important factor for the adrenal production of aldosterone. Many clinicians have assumed that prevention of angiotensin II (ATII) formation by the use of an ACE-I and/or blockade of the AT1-R by an ARB would therefore be effective in preventing the adrenal production of aldosterone. However, studies in the angiotensinogen knockout mouse, in which ATII is not present, have shown that modulation of serum sodium results in a significant increase in the adrenal production of aldosterone.[41] Although activation of the AT1-R is of importance for the adrenal production of aldosterone, other factors such as serum sodium and potassium levels are also of importance. ACE-I transiently suppresses aldosterone production, but, after several months, aldosterone levels rise back to or exceed baseline levels (aldosterone escape or aldosterone breakthrough).[42] Thus, no matter how much of an ACE-I and/or ARB is administered, the adrenal production of aldosterone over the long term cannot be prevented, and, as mentioned earlier, aldosterone plays an important blood pressure–independent effect on the progression of LVH. Furthermore, there is evidence that once the MR is activated by either aldosterone or cortisol, there is an upregulation of tissue ACE and of AT1-R expression,[43] resulting in a vicious cycle. Both ATII and aldosterone share some common signaling processes but also have independent signaling[44] such that it is necessary to block both ATII and the MR to have an optimal effect in preventing the development and progression of myocardial fibrosis and hypertrophy and thus the development of HF in patients with stage B HF. It is also important to point out that while MRAs block the effects of ATII-induced aldosterone production and subsequent development of myocardial fibrosis, they also block the effects of isoproterenol on myocardial fibrosis and injury.[45] Thus, it would seem that β-adrenergic activation, which is known to be of importance in the development of myocardial fibrosis, hypertrophy, and injury, is in part mediated by activation of the MR.

THE CHOICE OF AN MRA IN PATIENTS WITH STAGE B HF

Both spironolactone and eplerenone have been shown to block MRs and to reduce mortality in patients with HFREF. In patients with stage B HF with myocardial fibrosis and/or LVH due to hypertensive heart disease without the metabolic syndrome or diabetes mellitus, spironolactone would be the MR of choice because of the long familiarity with its use and its relatively low cost, except perhaps in young male patients and premenstrual women in whom eplerenone, because of its relatively greater specificity for the MR, is not associated with breast pain, gynecomastia in males, and menstrual irregularities in premenstrual women associated with the antiandrogen and prostagen effects of spironolactone. In patients with hypertensive heart disease and concomitant diabetes mellitus and/or visceral obesity, which predisposes to diabetes mellitus, eplerenone would seem to be the MRA of choice. Spironolactone has been found to increase HbA_{1c} levels and to worsen endothelial function in patients with diabetes mellitus,[46] whereas in those with HF without diabetes mellitus, it improves endothelial function, even on top of an ACE-I.[47] In a direct comparative study of spironolactone and eplerenone in patients with diabetes mellitus and HF,[48] spironolactone was shown to increase hemoglobin A1c levels, decrease adiponectin levels, and increase cortisol levels, whereas eplerenone did not. Eplerenone is considerably more expensive than spironolactone. However, it is now generic, at least in the United States, and its price can be expected to decrease, although not to the same level as spironolactone because of its more expensive synthesis.

LIMITATIONS TO THE USE OF AN MRA IN PATIENTS WITH STAGE B HF

Many patients with stage B HF are elderly and/or have concomitant diabetes mellitus and chronic renal disease, predisposing to hyperkalemia with the use of multiple RAAS inhibitors/blockers and, in particular, with an MRA. Patients with a serum potassium level greater than 5 mEq/L and those with an estimated glomerular filtration rate (eGFR) less than 30 mL/min/1.73 m^2 should not receive an MRA. It is necessary to obtain a serum potassium level measurement before initiation of an MRA and to serially monitor serum potassium and to adjust the dose of the MRA accordingly. In patients with normal renal function, serum potassium level should be measured within the first week after initiation of the MRA and then weekly for the first month. If the serum potassium level remains stable below 5 mEq/L, repeated measurements of serum potassium level can be obtained at routine follow-up visits. However, in patients with chronic kidney disease and/or diabetes mellitus, especially those with an eGFR less than 45 mL/min/1.73 m^2, measurement of serum potassium and renal function should be more frequent. If a change in electrolyte status is suspected, such as during an episode of diarrhea or vomiting, or when there is a change in medications that might affect serum potassium levels, such as an NSAID is added, measurement of serum potassium should be repeated. If at any time the serum potassium level is more than 5.5 mEq/L, the dose of MRA should be reduced by half, the measurement of serum potassium level repeated, and a careful review of the patients medications made. Patients may obtain NSAIDs over-the-counter without the physician's knowledge and therefore should be advised to avoid these medications and/or to promptly inform their physician if they take them. If the serum potassium level is 6 mEq/L or more in a nonhemolyzed blood sample and if there are electrocardiographic manifestations of hyperkalemia, the MRA should be discontinued and not be restarted until the serum potassium level is less than 5 mEq/L. The incidence of hyperkalemia in the major randomized trials of an MRA in patients with HFREF showing a reduction in total mortality[40] has been relatively low, and there has not been a single patient randomized to an MRA in these trials in which patient death has been attributed to hyperkalemia. However, in clinical practice where the inclusion and exclusion criteria used in the major randomized trials of MRAs have not been adhered to and/or when serum potassium level is not determined at baseline or serially monitored, there have been episodes of renal failure requiring dialysis and death. Thus, to obtain the benefits of an MRA as outlined earlier, it will be necessary for both the physician and patient to agree to serial monitoring of serum potassium.

SUMMARY

There is increasing evidence suggesting an important role of MRAs in the prevention of manifest HF (stage C and D HF) in patients with ACC/AHA stage B HF with myocardial fibrosis, LVH, and/or vascular stiffness. To achieve optimum benefits, it will be necessary to block both ATII and MR in order to carefully select patients and serially monitor serum potassium level and renal function. The proven benefits of MRAs in patients with chronic HFREF and HFREF after MI on total mortality and hospitalizations for HF hold the promise for the prevention of HF in patients with ACC/AHA stage B HF with a resultant reduction in mortality, morbidity, and health care costs. However, further prospective large-scale randomized studies in patients with stage B will be required before the risk/benefit of this strategy can be accurately assessed.

REFERENCES

1. Guder G, Bauersachs J, Frantz S, et al. Complementary and incremental mortality risk prediction by cortisol and aldosterone in chronic heart failure. Circulation 2007;115:1754–61.
2. Pitt B, Zannad F, Remme WJ, et al. The effect of spironolactone on morbidity and mortality in patients with severe heart failure. Randomized Aldactone Evaluation Study investigators. N Engl J Med 1999; 341:709–17.
3. Pitt B, Remme W, Zannad F, et al. Eplerenone, a selective aldosterone blocker, in patients with left ventricular dysfunction after myocardial infarction. N Engl J Med 2003;348:1309–21.
4. Zannad F, McMurray JJ, Krum H, et al. Eplerenone in patients with systolic heart failure and mild symptoms. N Engl J Med 2011;364:11–21.
5. Mottram PM, Haluska B, Leano R, et al. Effect of aldosterone antagonism on myocardial dysfunction in hypertensive patients with diastolic heart failure. Circulation 2004;110:558–65.
6. Pitt B, Bakris G, Ruilope LM, et al. Serum potassium and clinical outcomes in the eplerenone post-acute myocardial infarction heart failure efficacy and survival study (EPHESUS). Circulation 2008;118: 1643–50.
7. Tomaschitz A, Pilz S, Ritz E, et al. Plasma aldosterone levels are associated with increased cardiovascular mortality: the Ludwigshafen Risk and Cardiovascular Health (LURIC) study. Eur Heart J 2010;31:1237–47.
8. Beygui F, Vicaut E, Ecollan P, et al. Rationale for an early aldosterone blockade in acute myocardial infarction and design of the albatross trial. Am Heart J 2010;160:642–8.
9. Hunt SA, Abraham WT, Chin MH, et al. 2009 focused update incorporated into the ACC/AHA 2005 guidelines for the diagnosis and management of heart failure in adults. A report of the American College of Cardiology Foundation/American Heart Association Task Force on practice guidelines developed in collaboration with the International Society for Heart and Lung Transplantation. J Am Coll Cardiol 2009;53:e1–90.

10. Chapman N, Dobson J, Wilson S, et al. Effect of spironolactone on blood pressure in subjects with resistant hypertension. Hypertension 2007;49: 839–45.

11. Rossi GP, Sacchetto A, Visentin P, et al. Changes in left ventricular anatomy and function in hypertension and primary aldosteronism. Hypertension 1996;27: 1039–45.

12. Pitt B, Reichek N, Willenbrock R, et al. Effects of eplerenone, enalapril, and eplerenone/enalapril in patients with essential hypertension and left ventricular hypertrophy: the 4E-Left Ventricular Hypertrophy study. Circulation 2003;108:1831–8.

13. Savoia C, Touyz RM, Amiri F, et al. Selective mineralocorticoid receptor blocker eplerenone reduces resistance artery stiffness in hypertensive patients. Hypertension 2008;51:432–9.

14. Yoshida C, Goda A, Naito Y, et al. Role of plasma aldosterone concentration in regression of left-ventricular mass following antihypertensive medication. J Hypertens 2011;29:357–63.

15. Rocha R, Martin-Berger CL, Yang P, et al. Selective aldosterone blockade prevents angiotensin II/salt-induced vascular inflammation in the rat heart. Endocrinology 2002;143:4828–36.

16. Duprez D, De Buyzere M, Rietzchel E, et al. Inverse relationship between aldosterone and large artery compliance in chronically treated heart failure patients. Eur Heart J 1998;19:1371–6.

17. Brilla C. Renin-angiotensin-aldosterone system and myocardial fibrosis. Cardiovasc Res 2000;47:1–3.

18. Zannad F, Alla F, Dousset B, et al. Limitation of excessive extracellular matrix turnover may contribute to survival benefit of spironolactone therapy in patients with congestive heart failure: insights from the Randomized Aldactone Evaluation Study (RALES). RALES investigators. Circulation 2000;102:2700–6.

19. Martos R, Baugh J, Ledwidge M, et al. Diastolic heart failure: evidence of increased myocardial collagen turnover linked to diastolic dysfunction. Circulation 2007;115:888–95.

20. Ramires FJ, Mansur A, Coelho O, et al. Effect of spironolactone on ventricular arrhythmias in congestive heart failure secondary to idiopathic dilated or to ischemic cardiomyopathy. Am J Cardiol 2000;85: 1207–11.

21. Shah NC, Pringle SD, Donnan PT, et al. Spironolactone has antiarrhythmic activity in ischaemic cardiac patients without cardiac failure. J Hypertens 2007; 25:2345–51.

22. Rocha R, Funder JW. The pathophysiology of aldosterone in the cardiovascular system. Ann N Y Acad Sci 2002;970:89–100.

23. Callera GE, Touyz RM, Tostes RC, et al. Aldosterone activates vascular p38MAP kinase and NADPH oxidase via c-Src. Hypertension 2005;45:773–9.

24. Sam F, Xie Z, Ooi H, et al. Mice lacking osteopontin exhibit increased left ventricular dilation and reduced fibrosis after aldosterone infusion. Am J Hypertens 2004;17:188–93.

25. Usher MG, Duan SZ, Ivaschenko CY, et al. Myeloid mineralocorticoid receptor controls macrophage polarization and cardiovascular hypertrophy and remodeling in mice. J Clin Invest 2010;120: 3350–64.

26. Ito K, Hirooka Y, Sunagawa K. Acquisition of brain Na sensitivity contributes to salt-induced sympathoexcitation and cardiac dysfunction in mice with pressure overload. Circ Res 2009;104:1004–11.

27. Effect of enalapril on mortality and the development of heart failure in asymptomatic patients with reduced left ventricular ejection fractions. The SOLVD investigators. N Engl J Med 1992;327: 685–91.

28. Funder JW. RALES, EPHESUS and redox. J Steroid Biochem Mol Biol 2005;93:121–5.

29. Bocchi B, Kenouch S, Lamarre-Cliche M, et al. Impaired 11-beta hydroxysteroid dehydrogenase type 2 activity in sweat gland ducts in human essential hypertension. Hypertension 2004;43:803–8.

30. Pratt-Ubunama MN, Nishizaka MK, Boedefeld RL, et al. Plasma aldosterone is related to severity of obstructive sleep apnea in subjects with resistant hypertension. Chest 2007;131:453–9.

31. Goette A, Hoffmanns P, Enayati W, et al. Effect of successful electrical cardioversion on serum aldosterone in patients with persistent atrial fibrillation. Am J Cardiol 2001;88:906–9, A908.

32. Mosso LM, Carvajal CA, Maiz A, et al. A possible association between primary aldosteronism and a lower beta-cell function. J Hypertens 2007;25: 2125–30.

33. Stiefel P, Vallejo-Vaz A, Morillo S, et al. Role of the renin-angiotensin system and aldosterone on cardiometabolic syndrome. Int J Hypertens 2011;2011. DOI:10.4061/2011/685238. Article ID 685238, 8 pages.

34. Shibata S, Fujita T. The kidneys and aldosterone/mineralocorticoid receptor system in salt-sensitive hypertension. Curr Hypertens Rep 2011;13:109–15.

35. Pitt B. Plasma aldosterone levels in patients with coronary artery disease (CAD) without heart failure or myocardial infarction: implications for pathophsiology, prognosis, and therapy. Eur Heart J 2011. [Epub ahead of print].

36. Leopold JA, Dam A, Maron BA, et al. Aldosterone impairs vascular reactivity by decreasing glucose-6-phosphate dehydrogenase activity. Nat Med 2007;13:189–97.

37. Rajagopalan S, Duquaine D, King S, et al. Mineralocorticoid receptor antagonism in experimental atherosclerosis. Circulation 2002;105:2212–6.

38. Keidar S, Kaplan M, Pavlotzky E, et al. Aldosterone administration to mice stimulates macrophage

NADPH oxidase and increases atherosclerosis development: a possible role for angiotensin-converting enzyme and the receptors for angiotensin II and aldosterone. Circulation 2004;109: 2213–20.

39. Takai S, Jin D, Muramatsu M, et al. Eplerenone inhibits atherosclerosis in nonhuman primates. Hypertension 2005;46:1135–9.

40. Ezeckowitz J, McAllister F. Aldosterone blockade and left ventricular dysfunction: a systematic review of randomized clinical trials. Eur Heart J 2009;30(4): 469–77.

41. Okubo S, Niimura F, Nishimura H, et al. Angiotensin-independent mechanism for aldosterone synthesis during chronic extracellular fluid volume depletion. J Clin Invest 1997;99:855–60.

42. Struthers AD. The clinical implications of aldosterone escape in congestive heart failure. Eur J Heart Fail 2004;6:539–45.

43. Schiffrin EL. Effects of aldosterone on the vasculature. Hypertension 2006;47:312–8.

44. Min LJ, Mogi M, Li JM, et al. Aldosterone and angiotensin II synergistically induce mitogenic response in vascular smooth muscle cells. Circ Res 2005;97: 434–42.

45. Hori Y, Yoshioka K, Kanai K, et al. Spironolactone decreases isoproterenol-induced ventricular fibrosis and matrix metalloproteinase-2 in rats. Biol Pharm Bull 2011;34:61–5.

46. Davies JI, Band M, Morris A, et al. Spironolactone impairs endothelial function and heart rate variability in patients with type 2 diabetes. Diabetologia 2004; 47:1687–94.

47. Farquharson CA, Struthers AD. Spironolactone increases nitric oxide bioactivity, improves endothelial vasodilator dysfunction, and suppresses vascular angiotensin I/angiotensin II conversion in patients with chronic heart failure. Circulation 2000;101:594–7.

48. Yamaji M, Tsutamoto T, Kawahara C, et al. Effect of eplerenone versus spironolactone on cortisol and hemoglobin $A_1(c)$ levels in patients with chronic heart failure. Am Heart J 2010;160:915–21.

Nitric Oxide Modulation as a Therapeutic Strategy in Heart Failure

Anne L. Taylor, MD

KEYWORDS

- Nitric oxide • Heart failure • Oxidant stress

Nitric Oxide (NO) is recognized as one of the most important cardiovascular signaling molecules, with multiple regulatory effects on myocardial and vascular tissue as well as on other tissues and organ systems. Furchgott and Zawandski[1] first identified a substance secreted by endothelial cells that induced relaxation of vascular smooth muscle, which was initially called endothelium-derived relaxing factor (EDRF). EDRF was subsequently definitively identified as NO.[1–3] Though first recognized as a substance originating from endothelial cells that regulated vascular function and thrombogenicity, NO is also known to be expressed by cardiomyocytes as well as vascular endothelium, and to have multiple, complex regulatory roles on myocardial function including myocardial metabolism, mitochondrial respiration, autonomic function, contractility, relaxation, cell growth, ion channel behavior, and responsiveness to β-adrenergic stimulation, among others.[4–10] NO effects on the cardiovascular system and in heart failure may be positive or deleterious depending on the source of NO, the stimulus for NO release, the subcellular site of NO release, and the magnitude of NO release.[11–13]

In a wide range of cardiovascular diseases including systemic and pulmonary hypertension, coronary and peripheral atherosclerosis, ventricular hypertrophy, and right and left ventricular failure, there are significant alterations in NO bioavailability and signaling capacity.[6,14–24] With the growth in understanding of the range and mechanisms of NO effects on the cardiovascular system, it is now possible to consider pharmaceutical interventions that directly target either NO or key steps in NO effector pathways. This article briefly reviews some aspects of the cardiovascular effects of NO and abnormalities in NO regulation in heart failure, followed by a review of clinical trials of drugs that target specific aspects of NO signaling pathways.

GENERATION OF NITRIC OXIDE AND NITRIC OXIDE EFFECTOR PATHWAYS

NO is formed in tissues by the enzyme nitric oxide synthase (NOS), which converts L-arginine to L-citrulline and NO, and exists in myocardium in 3 different isoforms: neuronal NOS (nNOS or NOS1), endothelial NOS (eNOS or NOS3), and inducible NOS (iNOS or NOS2).[4–6,12,23] Nitric oxide synthases produce NO in response to different stimuli; for example, NOS1 and NOS3 require calcium for activation, whereas NOS2 does not. NOS2 is induced by proinflammatory cytokines and can release large quantities of NO, which can have direct toxic effects or increase the production of reactive oxygen species (ROS).[5,22,23] Quantities of NOS produced by each isoform may be quite

Funding support: None.

Disclosures: Dr Taylor received research support from Nitromed. She has been a consultant for Nitromed, CVRx, and the National Institutes of Health (NIH). She is currently a consultant for the NIH.

New York Presbyterian Hospital, Department of Medicine, Columbia University College of Physicians and Surgeons, 630 West 168th Street, Suite PH 1-132, New York, NY 10032, USA

E-mail address: ataylor@columbia.edu

Heart Failure Clin 8 (2012) 255–272

doi:10.1016/j.hfc.2011.11.002

different, and finally, NO produced by NOS may at times have quite different effects on myocardial function.[11,22,23] NOS isoforms are distributed within different cell compartments[12,13,22,23] and NO effects are determined in part by the specific subcellular target organelle, by the concentrations achieved within these cell compartments, and by the duration of time it is present.[5] The fact that NOS isoforms are located in different subcellular compartments and respond to different stimuli allows a heterogeneity of responses to a single molecule, NO, based on the specific cellular site of NO release, the isoform activated, and the stimulus for release, as well as the effector pathway activated.[6,12,22] **Table 1** summarizes some effects of activation of different NOS isoforms.

Two effector pathways for NO signaling are illustrated in **Fig. 1**. In endothelial cells, NOS converts L-arginine to L-citrulline and NO. NO then may bind to the heme moiety of soluble guanylyl cyclase (sGC), which catalyzes production of cyclic guanosine-3′,5′-monophosphate (cGMP) to activate protein kinases, ion channels, and cGMP-dependent phosphodiesterases.[4,5,23,25] cGMP effects are further regulated by degradation of GMP by phosphodiesterase type 5 (PDE-5). A second effector pathway for NO is cGMP independent and is the result of nitrosylation of cysteine residues (S-nitrosylation) of proteins.[25–29] Although the NO/cGMP signaling pathway was the first identified, S-nitrosylation is emerging as a widespread NO signaling mechanism with effects on cardiac excitation-contraction coupling, response to β-adrenergic stimulation, and arrhythmogenesis, to name a few.[25–29] Inactivation of the cGMP-derived NO effects occurs by degradation of cGMP by PDE-5, whereas the S-nitrosylation–dependent effects are regulated by protein denitrosylation.[22,29] Thus, biological effects of NO can occur by cGMP-dependent or cGMP-independent mechanisms, another variable that may contribute to the large number and heterogeneity of NO effects.

While NO is critical to the regulation of a large number of cellular functions, it can also be toxic

Table 1
Properties of NOS isoform activity in the normal and diseased heart

	NOS1 nNOS Neuronal NOS	NOS2 iNOS Inducible NOS	NOS3 eNOS Endothelial NOS
In Normal Hearts			
Antihypertrophic effect	✔		✔
Prohypertrophic effect		✔ or −	
Inhibition of L-type Ca^{2+} current	✔	−	✔
Net negative inotropic effect	✔	−	✔
Attenuate the β-adrenergic receptor-stimulated increase in myocardial contractility	✔		✔
Proapoptotic effect		✔ or −	
Profibrotic effect		✔ or −	
Induces left ventricular remodeling and failure		✔ or −	
During Hypertrophy/Failing/ Coronary Artery Occlusion			
Upregulated expression	✔	✔	
Downregulated expression			✔
Protects against remodeling	✔		✔
Protects against calcium overload	✔		
Limits infarct size		✔	
Improves contractile recovery after ischemia/reperfusion		✔	

From Umar S, van der Laarse A. Nitric oxide and nitric oxide synthase isoforms in the normal, hypertrophic, and failing heart. Mol Cell Biochem 2010;333(1–2):191–201; with permission.

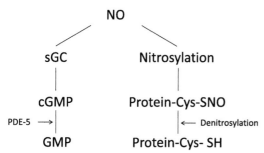

Fig. 1. Two signaling pathways for NO. NO activates soluble guanylyl cyclase (sGC), resulting in production of cyclic guanosine-3′,5′-monophosphate (cGMP) (cGMP). Phosphodiesterase type 5 (PDE-5) degrades cGMP. NO may also bind to the cysteine residue of proteins (S-nitrosylation), and deactivation occurs by denitrosylation.

through direct effects[5,22,23] or through the formation of ROS, for example, peroxynitrite, which can oxidize proteins that control contractility, ion channels, lipids in cell membranes, low-density lipoprotein (LDL), and nucleic acids. Peroxynitrite is also capable of inhibiting key steps in mitochondrial energy production.[5,23,30–33] In addition to ROS, reactive nitrogen species (RNS) can be generated and can contribute to the adverse effects of NO.[25,26,28] Other ROS generated by vascular and myocardial tissue including superoxide anion, hydrogen peroxide, and hydroxyl radical (generated by nicotinamide adenine dinucleotide phosphate oxidase, xanthine oxidase, and NOS3) in addition to peroxynitrate may influence the generation of NO or its effector capacity.[25,30,31] In healthy tissue, the balance between NO, ROS, and reactive nitrogen species (nitroso-redox balance) is such that favorable effects of NO predominate. By contrast, in states of excess ROS and RNS (high oxidant stress) the nitroso-redox balance shifts so that NO generation, bioavailability, and signaling capacity are impaired.

NITRIC OXIDE AND NITROSO-REDOX BALANCE IN HEART FAILURE

There is substantial evidence that NO dysregulation, endothelial dysfunction, and unfavorable changes in nitroso-redox balance occur in heart failure.[5,10,11,16–20,22–24,28,32–43] For example, there are data demonstrating that iNOS is induced by proinflammatory cytokines leading to the generation of toxic amounts of NO, which contribute to the formation of ROS and RNS as well as the accumulation of nitrosylated proteins.[15] iNOS (NOS2) is also associated with depression in myocardial contractility.[23,24] nNOS (NOS1) activity has also been found to be increased along with translocation of nNOS within failing hearts.[16] NO

bioavailability is affected by the presence of additional ROS such as superoxide, hydrogen peroxide, and hydroxyl radical. Further, NO generated by eNOS (NOS3), which has many cardioprotective properties, is reduced.[5,11,32,33] Changes in NOS activity, NO bioavailability, and nitroso-redox balance contribute to the vasoconstriction, depressed contractility, remodeling, electrophysiologic abnormalities, and altered metabolism of the failing heart.

Sharma and Davidoff[38] summarized evidence for abnormalities in NO bioavailability in heart failure, which include diminished NO release, increased inactivation of NO due to increased oxidant stress, and impaired antioxidant defenses leading to NO inactivation. Blunted endothelium-dependent flow-mediated dilation in response to acetylcholine infusion has been observed in patients with class III heart failure (both ischemic and nonischemic cardiomyopathies), consistent with diminished NO release.[17,36] Increased oxidant stress secondary to increased oxygen-derived free radicals is supported by the presence of elevated products of peroxidation generated by oxygen-derived free radicals in patients with advanced heart failure when compared with controls.[35,44,45] Diminished antioxidant capacity in heart failure has been suggested as another mechanism leading to greater oxidant stress and diminished endothelial function via more rapid inactivation of NO.[30,35,37]

Cardioprotection from postinfarction remodeling has been demonstrated in transgenic mice overexpressing NOS3,[46] whereas transgenic mice deficient in NOS3 developed more postinfarction remodeling, left ventricle (LV) dilatation, and functional impairment.[41,47,48] Postinfarction left ventricular remodeling and contractile function has been shown to be improved when eNOS activity is pharmacologically enhanced.[49,50]

NITRIC OXIDE AS A THERAPEUTIC TARGET IN HEART FAILURE

In the context of impairment in NO bioavailability, altered NO signaling capacity, elevation in oxidant stress, and an unfavorable nitroso-redox balance in heart failure, enhancement of NO availability, improvement in NO signaling, or a more favorable shift in nitroso-redox balance have potential as therapeutic targets to improve outcomes in heart failure. At present there are 3 types of pharmacologic agents that specifically target NO bioavailability or signaling that have been tested in heart failure trials. Two of these agents target different points in the NO-sGC-cGMP effector pathway, whereas the actions of the third are based on the ability to release NO on biotransformation, and thus may act via either effector pathway. These agents include: (1) organonitrates, which must undergo biotransformation or dissociation to release NO; (2) agents that target sGC independently of NO and act synergistically to increase the sensitivity of sGC to NO or to directly stimulate sGC completely independently of NO; and (3) PDE-5 inhibitors, which diminish the degradation of cGMP thereby prolonging NO effects.

NITRIC OXIDE DONORS

Organonitrate-induced vasodilation has been recognized for more than a century and has been exploited clinically to decrease cardiac filling pressure and improve coronary blood flow. Drugs that release NO may spontaneously release it under physiologic conditions (nitroprusside, NO gas) or require biotransformation for the release of NO (nitroglycerin, isosorbide dinitrate).[51] NO then activates NO effector pathways as summarized in **Fig. 1**.[3,51–53] The precise mechanism of nitrate biotransformation has not been completely characterized, but recent evidence suggests that mitochondrial aldehyde dehydrogenase is, in part, responsible for the biotransformation of nitroglycerin.[52–55] Although nitrates were used primarily for their hemodynamic properties and their effects on the microcirculation,[56] it was also noted that long-term therapy resulted in blunting of their hemodynamic effects, a phenomenon described as nitrate tolerance.[54,57–59] In addition, endothelial function measured by change in forearm blood flow in response to acetylcholine[59,60] was also impaired by long-term therapy, supporting loss of NO-mediated effects with prolonged exposure. While nitroglycerin is the prototypical organonitrate, it is of interest that there may be differences in the biological effects of different esters of nitroglycerin.[60,61] Although the biology of nitrate tolerance remains controversial, mitochondrial aldehyde dehydrogenase–2 is thought to play a role, in part, via formation of mitochondrial ROS,[57,58,62] resulting in NO inactivation. Tolerance may also be the result of the oxidation of the heme moiety of sGC, rendering it insensitive to NO or to reduction in nitroglycerine biotransformation by mitochondrial aldehyde dehydrogenase, along with a concurrent increased mitochondrial production of ROS.[57]

Consistent prevention of the development of tolerance clinically with antioxidants such as vitamin C or acetylcysteine and angiotensin-converting enzyme inhibitors (ACE-Is) has been unsuccessful.[63–65] However, it was noted that the addition of the smooth muscle relaxant hydralazine to nitrate-treated aortic rings was effective in diminishing the development of tolerance.[66] In addition to its effects on vascular smooth muscle relaxation, hydralazine has been shown to have potent antioxidant effects mediated in part by inhibition of reduced nicotinamide adenine dinucleotide oxidase, with reduced formation of peroxynitrite and superoxide anion,[67,68] as well as inhibition of NOS2 gene expression.[69] In animal models of heart failure[68,70] as well as human studies of patients with congestive heart failure,[71] concomitant administration of hydralazine with organonitrates resulted in prolongation of hemodynamic effects of nitrates without development of tolerance. Bauer and Fung[70] showed sustained reduction in left ventricular end-diastolic pressure and left ventricular systolic pressure when hydralazine was added to nitroglycerin treatment of rats with congestive heart failure. Gogia and colleagues,[71] in a clinical study, similarly found that the addition of hydralazine to nitrate infusion resulted in sustained reduction in mean pulmonary artery pressure, mean pulmonary wedge pressure, and mean arterial pressure compared with treatment with nitrate infusion only. **Fig. 2** demonstrates the proposed impact of combined hydralazine and nitrates on NO production and nitroso-redox balance.

The effect of the combination of hydralazine and isosorbide dinitrate on outcomes in patients with heart failure was first tested 25 years ago in the Vasodilator in Heart Failure I (V-HeFT I) trial.[72] In this trial, which preceded the discovery of NO, the therapeutic target was the hemodynamic effect of balanced reduction in cardiac filling pressures and systemic vascular resistance. The trial was based on use of an oral regimen that would reproduce the hemodynamic effects of intravenous nitroprusside, rather than effects on NO, which had not yet been discovered. Six hundred male patients with class II to IV heart failure, treated only with digoxin and diuretics, were randomized to 1 of 3 treatment arms: hydralazine plus isosorbide dinitrate (ISDN/HYD), prazocin, an α-blocker with similar hemodynamic effects to ISDN/HYD, and placebo, with mortality as the end point. Whereas the hemodynamic profile of the 2 vasodilator interventions were not very different, the mortality outcome did differ (**Fig. 3**). Mortality curves for placebo and prazocin were superimposable, whereas that of ISDN/HYD demonstrated superiority in survival. The difference was maintained throughout the trial with a P value of 0.06 at the end of the trial. Though not quite reaching statistical significance, the outcome nonetheless was a sentinel one, as it strongly suggested that properties other than the hemodynamic effects of vasodilators

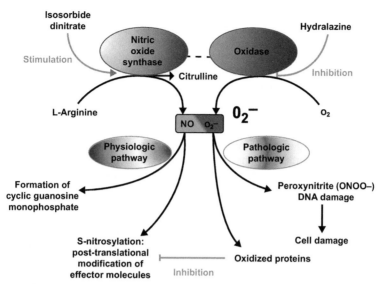

Fig. 2. Consequences of NO and superoxide balance disruption in heart failure patients. (*From* Hare JM. Nitroso-redox balance in the cardiovascular system. N Engl J Med 2004;351:2113; with permission.)

could have a mortality benefit, and importantly that the hemodynamic effects of drugs could not be used as a surrogate for mortality benefit. Subsequently, the second vasodilator in heart failure trial, V-HeFT II,[73] which compared the ACE-I enalapril with ISDN/HYD, showed enalapril to confer better survival; however, as there was no placebo group comparison of the 2 agents with placebo was not available.

The discoveries of NO, the mechanism of action of organonitrates, and the expansion of knowledge regarding the possible role of NO in normal and diseased cardiovascular states occurred after the V-HeFT trials, but provided a possible rationale for the differences in outcomes of treatment groups observed in V-HeFT I.

The two V-HeFT trials included an all-male cohort; however, the ethnic make-up of the cohort was serendipitously about 30% African American, thus providing an opportunity, post hoc, to assess whether there were differences in drug response by ethnicity. The rationale for such an analysis was based on the lesser antihypertensive effects of ACE-Is as monotherapy for hypertension in African

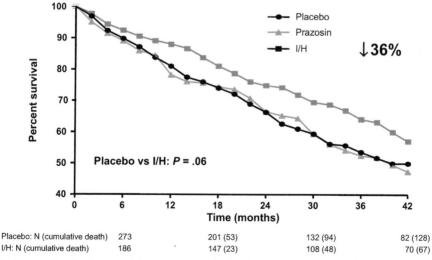

Fig. 3. Survival curves for the 3 arms of the V-HeFT I trial. Placebo and prazosin had identical outcomes, whereas isosorbide dinitrate hydralazine (I/H) improved survival. (*From* Cohn JN, Archibald DG, Ziesche S, et al. Effect of vasodilator therapy on mortality in chronic congestive heart failure. Results of a Veterans Administration Cooperative Study. N Engl J Med 1986;314(24):1547–52; with permission.)

Americans[74] as well as differences in responsiveness to ACE-Is in African Americans with heart failure in the SOLVD treatment and prevention trials.[75] Post hoc analysis of the outcomes by ethnicity revealed that African Americans derived greater benefit from the combination of ISDN/HYD (**Fig. 4**).[76] These data provided the context for the hypothesis for the African American Heart Failure Trial (A-HeFT), the first randomized trial of combined NO donor and antioxidant targeting enhancement of NO bioavailability, rather than the hemodynamic effects of these drugs.[77,78]

The A-HeFT trial[77,78] assessed the effect of combined ISDN/HYD (with nitrates as NO donor and hydralazine as antioxidant) on cardiovascular outcomes in African American patients with advanced heart failure. Self-identified African American patients with dilated LVs and low ejection fractions, treated with background neurohormonal antagonists (93% ACE-I/angiotensin-receptor blocker, 39% spironolactone, 87% β-blockers, 62% digoxin) were randomized to receive added placebo or fixed-dose combined ISDN/HYD, and were followed for 18 months. The primary end point was a score that weighted death, first heart failure hospitalization, and quality of life at 6 months. The trial was stopped early by its data safety monitoring board because of a highly significant mortality benefit in the fixed-dose ISDN/HYD group (**Fig. 5**A). Death, first heart failure hospitalization, and improvement in quality of life were all significantly improved by added fixed-dose ISDN/HYD (see **Fig. 5**B).

Forty percent of the A-HeFT cohort comprised women, thus providing the only randomized clinical trial data on outcomes in women treated with combined ISDN/HYD.[79] Post hoc analysis comparing women with men revealed the following. Although there were no differences by sex in background medications, baseline clinical characteristics significantly differed in some categories; men had more renal insufficiency, atrial fibrillation, and slightly lower qualifying ejection fractions, whereas women had more diabetes, lower hemoglobins, and slightly higher blood pressures, but worse quality-of-life scores. Outcomes were directionally similar for men and women. Though women appeared to have a greater mortality benefit, no sex-by-treatment interaction in this retrospective analysis was observed.

Comparison of outcomes by age greater than or less than age 65 years (Taylor and colleagues, unpublished data, 2010) revealed similar outcomes in the 2 age groups, despite those older than age 65 being significantly less likely to be treated with background neurohormonal antagonists. An interesting synergy between ISDN/HYD

and aldosterone antagonism was suggested by a significantly improved mortality in those treated with both agents,[80] consistent with an improvement in NO-mediated vascular responses with spironolactone treatment.[81] Significant improvement on echocardiographic ejection fraction and decrease in left ventricular diastolic diameter at 6 months[82] was evident in the ISDN/HYD treatment arm. The incidence of atrial fibrillation was also decreased in the treated group.[83]

An important treatment effect of fixed-dose ISDN/HYD was a significant decrease of 2 to 5 mm Hg in systolic blood pressure and a 2- to 4-mm Hg reduction in diastolic blood pressure.[78,84] However, beneficial effects of fixed-dose ISDN/HYD were similar in patients with blood pressures above and below the group median blood pressure.[84] Therefore, blood pressure reduction was likely not the cause of the improved outcomes. This proposal is supported by findings from other clinical trials on heart failure whereby blood pressure was lowered by pharmacologic treatment, with no mortality benefit observed.[72,85,86]

The conclusion from the A-HeFT trial was that there was a significant and consistent improvement in mortality, hospitalization, event-free survival, and quality of life in a selected population with advanced heart failure, likely via an additional or alternative mechanistic pathway to those addressed by neurohormonal blockade. The evidence for nitrates as NO donors,[52–55] for hydralazine as antioxidant,[67–69] and for a favorable interaction between the two[66,68,70,71] strongly suggest that enhanced NO bioavailability and/or improved oxidant stress played a role in the positive outcomes of the V-HeFT and A-HeFT trials.

Further studies will be required to precisely identify the mechanism of action of the combination, to understand population variables determining response and other pathophysiologic states in which there might be benefit, and to explore possible synergies with other agents used in therapy for heart failure.

SOLUBLE GUANYLYL CYCLASE AS A TARGET FOR TREATMENT OF HEART FAILURE

The desire for the pharmacologic ability to activate sGC independently of NO, under conditions when sGC is likely to be unresponsive to NO, as well as to circumvent the problem of tolerance associated with organonitrates, has contributed to the development of drugs that directly target activation of sGC.

NO activation of sGC may occur either by in vivo generation of NO by NOS or via exogenous administration of inhaled NO gas or by administration of drugs such as organonitrates, which release NO

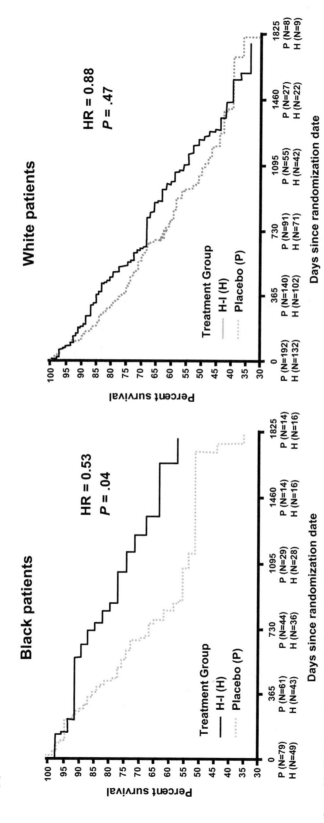

Fig. 4. (A, B) Retrospective analysis of mortality differences between black and white patients with heart failure, treated with combined isosorbide dinitrate/hydralazine or enalapril in V-HeFT I (A) and V-HeFT II (B). These observations formed the basis for the hypothesis of the African American Heart Failure Trial. (*From* Carson P, Ziesche S, Johnson G, et al. Racial differences in response to therapy for heart failure: analysis of the vasodilator-heart failure trials. Vasodilator-Heart Failure Trial Study Group. J Cardiac Fail 1999;5:178–87; with permission.)

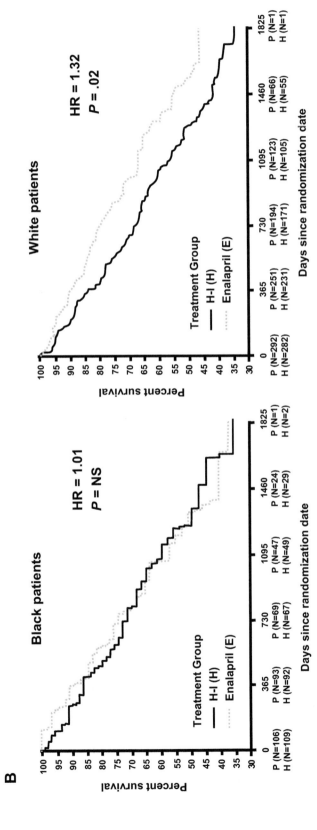

Fig. 4. (continued)

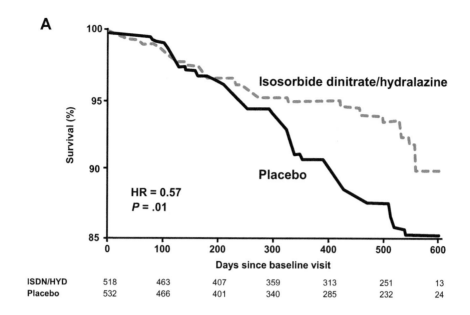

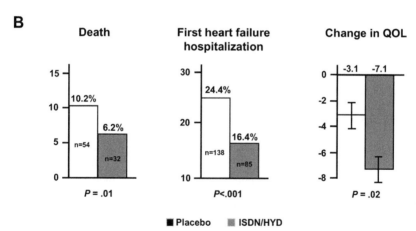

■ Placebo   ▨ ISDN/HYD

Fig. 5. (*A, B*). Kaplan-Meier survival curves (*A*) and outcomes (*B*) in the 2 treatment arms of the African American Heart Failure Trial. Patients were randomized to fixed-dose combined isosorbide dinitrate/hydralazine (ISDN/HYD) or placebo added to neurohormone blockade. HR, hazard ratio; QOL, quality of life. (*From* Taylor AL, Ziesche S, Yancy C, et al. Combination of isosorbide dinitrate and hydralazine in blacks with heart failure. N Engl J Med 2004;351(20):2052; with permission.)

on biotransformation (**Fig. 6**). An important feature of the activation of sGC by NO is the requirement that the heme moiety of sGC be in its reduced state (Fe^{2+}). Under conditions of high oxidant stress, the heme moiety of sGC may become oxidized (Fe^{3+}), which renders sGC unresponsive to NO.[87–91]

Direct activators of sGC (see **Fig. 6**) comprise a group of pharmacologic agents that can activate the sGC → cGMP → protein kinase pathway independently of NO, thus producing NO effects when NO is either unavailable or unable to activate this signaling pathway. In 1994, Ko and colleagues[92] described a compound that directly stimulated

platelet sGC and sensitized sGC to NO. In 2001, Stasch and colleagues[93] identified a site on sGC that was stimulated by a compound, Bay 41-2272, resulting in NO-like effects including increased platelet cGMP levels, inhibition of platelet aggregation, and decreased blood pressure in a rat model of hypertension. Bay 41-2272 was also found to produce decreased blood pressure when administered orally[93] and, importantly, there were no signs of tolerance to these effects. Of interest, survival was also significantly improved in hypertensive rats treated with Bay 41-2272.[93]

Subsequent studies summarized by Boerrigter and Burnett[91,94,95] demonstrated that the compound

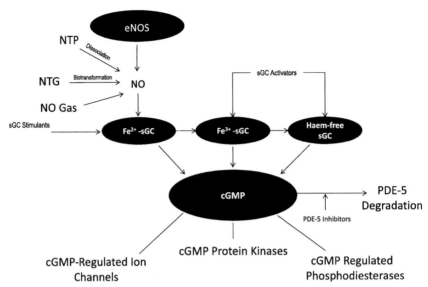

Fig. 6. NO signaling via the cGMP pathway. Drugs specifically targeting NO modulation in heart failure have included agents that release NO, agents activating sGC, and those inhibiting the degradation of cGMP. NTG, nitroglycerin; NTP, nitroprusside.

was synergistic with NO, reduced renal vascular and systematic vascular resistance, and increased cardiac output. A limitation of this compound was that it did not activate sGC with an oxidized heme moiety or the heme-free form of sGC.

Subsequently Stasch and colleagues[96] identified a similar compound (Bay 58-2667), which activated sGC in an NO-independent manner, as opposed to the NO synergistic way described for Bay 41-2272. Bay 58-2667 activated the oxidized and heme-deficient forms of sGC, which were insensitive to NO and to Bay 41-2272. The compound was found to produce NO-like effects (eg, inhibition of platelet aggregation, vasorelaxation), even in the presence of induced nitrate tolerance.[96] The hemodynamic effects of the compound on veins and arteries were similar to nitroglycerin, with the significant advantage that tolerance did not occur and that it was effective in the state of induced nitrate tolerance.

These 2 compounds were the first of a class of agents that directly targeted the sGC step in the cGMP-dependent activation of NO, suggesting the possibility of activation of NO signaling in a more specific way than NO donation, and in settings of endothelial dysfunction and nitrate tolerance.

Currently available activators of sGC that have been tested clinically may be subdivided, based on whether they are able to activate oxidized or

heme-free sGC (see **Fig. 6**). Those agents that require the presence of sGC containing the reduced heme moiety (Bay 41-2272, riociquat), and those that stimulate sGC synergistically with NO but are incapable of activating oxidized or heme-free sGC, are called sGC stimulators; those agents capable of directly activating oxidized or heme-free sGC that is insensitive to NO (Bay 58-2667, cinaciguat) are designated sGC activators.[87,89,91,93–95]

There is substantial evidence for impairment in the NO-sGC-cGMP signal pathway in hypertension, heart failure, and atherosclerosis.[97–100] Of importance, treatment with both sGC stimulators and sGC activators[91,94–96,99,101–104] in experimental models of hypertension and heart failure as well as pulmonary hypertension have demonstrated positive hemodynamic effects in response to both of these types of agent. In a canine model of tachycardia-induced heart failure, the sGC stimulator (Bay 41-2272) decreased systemic and pulmonary vascular resistance, increased cardiac output, and maintained renal blood flow as well as urine output. However, right atrial pressure was not decreased.[94,98] Of significance is that activation of the renin-angiotensin-aldosterone system, an important side effect of diuretic therapy in heart failure, did not occur.

Using Bay 58-2667, an sGC activator that is both NO-independent and heme-independent, in the same model of tachycardia-induced canine heart failure, Boerrigter and colleagues[95] found that mean arterial, pulmonary arterial, and pulmonary capillary wedge pressures as well as right atrial pressure were reduced, whereas cardiac output and renal blood flow were increased. Plasma renin and aldosterone levels did not increase, nor was tolerance to drug effect observed.

Based on these experimental findings, a clinical trial examined the hemodynamic responses to the direct activator of sGC, cinaciguat (Bay 58-2667) in patients with acute decompensated heart failure.[105] The study was a nonrandomized, uncontrolled assessment of hemodynamics, safety, and tolerability of the drug. The investigators found that a 6-hour infusion of the drug resulted in significant reductions in pulmonary capillary wedge pressure, mean right atrial pressure, mean pulmonary arterial pressure, and pulmonary and systemic vascular resistance, with a significant increase in cardiac output. The proportion of patients responding to the drug increased with increasing duration of infusion; after 6 hours, 90% of patients had responded. The most common side effect reported was hypotension. In pharmacokinetics and pharmacodynamics studies,[106] there was a rapid decline in plasma concentration of drug as well as resolution of hemodynamic effects at termination of the infusion. The effects of the sGC stimulator, Bay 65-2521, also called riociguat, which stimulates sGC independently of NO as well as synergistically with low concentrations of NO, has been examined in patients with pulmonary hypertension. Grimminger and colleagues[107] described the acute hemodynamic effects of oral riociguat in patients with pulmonary hypertension (pulmonary vascular resistance >300 dyn/s/cm^5) associated with chronic thromboembolic pulmonary hypertension, interstitial lung disease, or primary pulmonary artery hypertension. The investigators found significant reductions in pulmonary arterial pressures, pulmonary vascular resistance, and systemic vascular resistance, and increases in cardiac index. Ghofrani and colleagues[102] reported favorable effects on pulmonary hemodynamics and exercise capacity in 72 patients with pulmonary hypertension treated over 12 weeks with riociguat. Further clinical trials of patients with pulmonary hypertension are in progress (clinicaltrials.gov).

Although investigation of the full impact of these drugs on heart failure is at an early stage, the favorable hemodynamic effects, the absence of the development of tolerance or further activation of the renin-angiotensin-aldosterone system, the ability to be effective in disease states with high oxidant stress, and the favorable pharmacodynamics are strong indicators of a future role in the treatment of heart failure.

PDE-5 INHIBITION IN SYSTOLIC HEART FAILURE

Another control point in the NO-sGC-cGMP signaling pathway is the interaction between cGMP and catabolic cGMP phosphodiesterases (see **Fig. 6**). Phosphodiesterases are a family of enzymes that differ by structure, substrate used, tissue location, expression, and response to specific inhibitors.[108–110] PDE-5 is a phosphodiesterase associated with the degradation of cGMP and thus plays an important regulatory role in NO-mediated effects. PDE-5 expression has been found to be highest in lung tissue, platelets, and vascular smooth muscle, is specific for cGMP as substrate, and when bound to cGMP results in degradation of cGMP and diminished NO effects.[108–110] Thus, inhibitors of PDE-5 should amplify and prolong NO effects.

Because of the high PDE-5 levels found in lung tissue as well as the upregulation of PDE-5 observed in states associated with pulmonary hypertension, including pulmonary hypertension associated with left heart failure, PDE-5 inhibitors were first tested in pulmonary hypertension.[111,112] Decreased pulmonary artery pressures and improved functional capacity were noted in these studies.[111,112]

In normal myocytes, PDE-5 expression is low and thus its role in normal myocyte physiology is not clear. However, in cardiac disease states, including pulmonary hypertension, right ventricular hypertrophy, and failure, PDE-5 has been found to be upregulated,[108–110,113–115] and the resultant greater degradation of cGMP may contribute to the impairment NO-mediated vasomotor and vascular remodeling effects in these conditions. PDE-5 has been found has been found to be increased in hypertrophied right ventricular myocardium[114] but not to be expressed in normal right ventricles. The same investigators[114] found that PDE-5 inhibition in hypertrophied, but not normal, right ventricular myocardium resulted in increased contractility and increases in cGMP levels.

Lu and colleagues[113] found that the increase in PDE-5 expression correlated with markers of oxidative stress in myocardial samples from patients with end-stage heart failure. This group also measured elevated levels of PDE-5 in left ventricular tissue from mice with aortic constriction–induced left ventricular hypertrophy and failure, and found that pharmacologic attenuation of oxidative stress resulted in decreased PDE-5 protein and activity in the mice hearts.[113] Takimoto and colleagues[116] demonstrated that the PDE-5 inhibitor sildenafil prevented the development of myocardial hypertrophy and improved left ventricular function in a murine model of pressure overload left ventricular hypertrophy. Nagayama and colleagues[117] found that sildenafil also prevented progressive remodeling in the same murine model of developed and long-standing left ventricular pressure overload hypertrophy. Lewis and colleagues[118] tested pretreatment with sildenafil as prevention of isoproterenol-induced hypertrophy in rat hearts. Sildenafil pretreatment effectively prevented isoproterenol-induced hypertrophy, improved survival, and resulted in significantly increased myocardial tissue levels of cGMP. While studies suggest that PDE-5 may play a minor role in cGMP balance in the normal left ventricular myocardium, it may nonetheless be important in the pressure-overloaded and failing left ventricular myocardium. Pokreisz and colleagues[115] found

that PDE-5 expression was greater in LVs from patients with dilated cardiomyopathies.

Because pulmonary hypertension associated with left ventricular failure confers a worse prognosis, is a major contributor to the diminished functional capacity in heart failure, and previous studies demonstrated efficacy in improving hemodynamics and functional capacity in patients with pulmonary hypertension, several trials have been conducted to assess the impact of PDE-5 inhibitors in the setting of left ventricular failure including some patients with associated pulmonary hypertension (**Table 2**).[118–123]

Lewis and colleagues[118] reported hemodynamic and functional data from 13 patients with left heart failure treated with sildenafil. These investigators examined right heart hemodynamics, gas exchange, and right ventricular function at rest

Table 2
Summary of clinical trials of PDE-5 inhibitors in left heart failure

Study Reference	Inclusion Criteria	N	Drug	Duration	First End Point	Additional End Points	Outcomes
Lewis et al[118]	NYHA III LVEF <0.35	13	Sildenafil	Acute single dose	ΔPeak V_{O_2}	ΔΔLVEF, RVEF Serum lactate Hemodynamics VE/V_{CO_2}	↓PAP, ↑PVR ↑RVEF, ↑CI ↑Peak V_{O_2} nc LVEF nc MAP
Lewis et al[120]	NYHA II–IV LVEF<0.35, mPAP>25	34	Sildenafil	12 wk	ΔPeak V_{O_2}	Hemodynamics ΔLVEF, RVEF ΔQoL, 6MW test	↑Peak V_{O_2} ↑RVEF ↑CO, nc PCWP ↑ QoL ↑ 6MW distance nc MAP, nc HR
Guazzi et al[123]	NYHA II–III LVEF <0.35 Age <65	46	Sildenafil	6 mo	ΔPeak V_{O_2} ΔVE/V_{CO_2}	ΔErgo reflex ΔFMD Hemodynamics	↑Peak V_{O_2} ↑FMD ↓VE/V_{CO_2} ↓PASP
Behling et al[122]	NYHA I–III LVEF <0.4	19	Sildenafil	4 wk	ΔPeak V_{O_2} ΔEcho PASP	ΔVE/V_{CO_2} FMD	↑Peak V_{O_2} ↓VE/V_{CO_2} ↓PASP nc FMD
Guazzi et al[124]	NYHA II–III LVEF <0.40 LV diastolic dysfunction All male	45	Sildenafil	1 y	ΔPeak V_{O_2} ΔLVEF	LA + LV size LVEF PASP Mitral E/A E/E' QoL	↑LVEF ↑Peak V_{O_2} ↑QoL ↓VE/V_{CO_2} ↓E/A ↓E/E'

↑, increase; ↓, decrease; nc, no change.

Abbreviations: 6MW, 6-minute walking; CI, cardiac index; CO, cardiac output; E/A, ratio between early (E) and late (atrial, A) ventricular filling velocity; E/E', ratio of mitral peak velocity of early filling (E) to early diastolic mitral annular velocity; FMD, flow-mediated dilation; HR, heart rate; LA, left atrium; LV, left ventricle; LVEF, left ventricular ejection fraction; MAP, mean arterial pressure; mPAP, mean pulmonary arterial pressure; NYHA, New York Heart Association class; PAP, pulmonary arterial pressure; PASP, pulmonary artery systolic pressure; PCWP, pulmonary capillary wedge pressure; PVR, pulmonary vascular resistance; RVEF, right ventricular ejection fraction; QoL, quality of life; V_{CO_2}, carbon dioxide production; VE, ventilatory efficiency; V_{O_2}, oxygen uptake.

and with exercise following acute administration of 50 mg sildenafil. Results of the study showed that sildenafil significantly reduced resting pulmonary arterial pressure, pulmonary vascular resistance, and systemic vascular resistance, while increasing resting and exercise cardiac index. With exercise, pulmonary arterial pressure, pulmonary vascular resistance, and the ratio of pulmonary vascular resistance to systemic vascular resistance were reduced significantly. Peak oxygen uptake (Vo_2) and ventilatory efficiency also significantly improved. Of note, in this small clinical study improvements in hemodynamics and exercise capacity were limited to patients with pulmonary hypertension. In a second study, Lewis and colleagues[120] studied outcomes of 34 patients with systolic heart failure and secondary pulmonary hypertension who were treated with sildenafil. Patients without pulmonary hypertension were excluded based on findings from their first study. Subjects were randomized to 12 weeks of treatment with sildenafil or placebo. Exercise capacity, quality of life, and hemodynamic data were collected. In the sildenafil group, during cardiopulmonary exercise testing there was a significant improvement in peak Vo_2, a significant reduction in pulmonary vascular resistance, and a significant increase in cardiac output, without any impact on pulmonary capillary wedge pressure, mean arterial pressure, heart rate, or systemic vascular resistance. Quality-of-life scores and the 6-minute walking test also significantly improved in the sildenafil group.

In a longer-term study, Guazzi and colleagues[123] randomized 46 patients with class II to III heart failure of ischemic or idiopathic origin to either sildenafil or placebo for 6 months. The presence or absence of pulmonary hypertension was not defined. Data were collected to measure pulmonary hemodynamics, ventilation capacity, and brachial artery flow-mediated dilation (to test for the therapeutic impact on an NO-mediated process) at 3 and 6 months. After 6 months on sildenafil, patients showed significant improvements in exercise ventilation and aerobic efficiency, as well as improved brachial artery flow-mediated dilation. Of importance, neither heart rate nor systemic vascular resistance changed in the 2 groups. Behling and colleagues[122] found similar outcomes in 19 patients with decreased left ventricular function, treated over a 4-week period. Significant improvements in functional capacity, ventilatory efficiency, and pulmonary hypertension were found. Of interest, no change in brachial artery flow-mediated dilation was noted in the sildenafil group in this study; however, the sample size was smaller and the duration of treatment was shorter in

comparison with the group studied by Guazzi and colleagues.[123]

In a subsequent study, Guazzi and colleagues[124] examined a cohort of 45 male patients with systolic heart failure randomized to either sildenafil or placebo for 12 months. Left ventricular ejection fraction, echocardiographic parameters of diastolic filling, cardiopulmonary exercise capacity, and quality of life were measured. At 12 months, ejection fraction, left ventricular volume index (ml/m^2), left ventricular mass index (g/m^2), and left ventricular end-diastolic volume index (ml/m^2) all significantly decreased, suggesting an effect on left ventricular remodeling. Pulmonary artery systolic pressure decreased significantly in the sildenafil group while peak Vo_2 during cardiopulmonary exercise testing increased significantly. Quality of life significantly improved in the sildenafil group, as did echocardiographic parameters of ventricular filling. Of interest, this group was not limited to patients with associated pulmonary hypertension, and the cohort was well treated with background ACE-Is and β-blockers, suggesting that additional benefit might be derived from the addition of this treatment to currently recommended therapies for heart failure. However, larger trials of longer duration are necessary to determine whether there is a mortality effect in addition to the positive hemodynamic and functional effects.

In summary, PDE-5 inhibitors may have a therapeutic role in patients with left ventricular systolic dysfunction, particularly when secondary pulmonary hypertension is associated with left ventricular dysfunction. However, the studies of Guazzi and colleagues[123,124] suggest that benefit may occur even without defined pulmonary hypertension. Longer-term effects on mortality and morbidity in large, diverse cohorts will be of considerable interest.

SUMMARY

NO has emerged as a very important cardiovascular regulatory molecule, with numerous important direct myocardial effects mediated by activation of cGMP or by nitrosylation of cysteine residues on proteins. NO can be generated by 3 different NO synthases located in different cell compartments that respond to different stimuli for release of NO, and which are capable of releasing amounts of NO that considerably differ quantitatively. These properties account for the large quantity and heterogeneity of actions of a single signaling molecule. NO effects on cardiovascular tissue may be positive or deleterious, depending on the NOS source of NO, the cell compartment into which NO is released, and the quantity released, as well as the cellular redox state. Evidence suggests that endothelial-derived NO bioavailability and/or signaling capacity is impaired in heart failure, and that drugs which increase the bioavailability or activity of endothelial derived NO may have beneficial effects on myocardial function, morbidity, and mortality. At present there are 3 types of drugs that directly affect NO bioavailability or signaling capacity that have demonstrated positive clinical outcomes in heart failure: organonitrates combined with hydralazine, soluble guanylyl cyclase stimulants/activators, and PDE-5 inhibitors. Mortality and morbidity as well as the hemodynamics of heart failure have been favorably affected by combined nitrates and hydralazine, while sGC stimulators/activators have demonstrated promising hemodynamic and functional effects without the tolerance observed with nitrates. Finally, PDE-5 inhibitors have favorable effects on right ventricular function and pulmonary hemodynamics, ventilatory efficiency, exercise capacity, and quality of life in patients with heart failure.

The early twenty-first century may well be the period in which we understand and exploit the NO signaling pathway as a therapeutic target for cardiovascular diseases. Agents such as NO donors, nitroso-modulating agents, sGC stimulant/activators, and PDE-5 inhibitors can affect NO signaling at different points in the NO effector pathways. It is the case that heart failure syndrome is a final common pathway of a heterogeneous group of diseases with prominent dysregulation of NO as well as the better studied neurohormonal abnormalities. It may well be that NO dysregulation in heart failure is a similarly heterogeneous process, thus supporting the ongoing study of multiple NO-modulating agents.

REFERENCES

1. Furchgott RF, Zawadzki JV. The obligatory role of endothelial cells in the relaxation of arterial smooth muscle by acetylcholine. Nature 1980;288(5879): 373–6.
2. Moncada S, Herman AG, Vanhoutte P. Endothelium-derived relaxing factor is identified as nitric oxide. Trends Pharmacol Sci 1987;8(10):365–8.
3. Ignarro LJ. Nitric oxide: a unique endogenous signaling molecule in vascular biology. Biosci Rep 1999;19(2):51–71.
4. Loscalzo J, Welch G. Nitric oxide and its role in the cardiovascular system. Prog Cardiovasc Dis 1995; 38(2):87–104.
5. Pacher P, Beckman JS, Liaudet L, et al. Nitric oxide and peroxynitrite in health and disease. Physiol Rev 2007;87(1):315–424.
6. Massion PB, Feron O, Dessy C, et al. Nitric oxide and cardiac function: ten years after, and continuing. Circ Res 2003;93(5):388–98.
7. Moens AL, Yang R, Watts VL, et al. Beta 3-adrenor eceptor regulation of nitric oxide in the cardiovascular system. J Mol Cell Cardiol 2010; 48(6):1088–95.
8. Moncada S, Palmer RM, Higgs EA. Nitric oxide: physiology, pathophysiology, and pharmacology. Pharmacol Rev 1991;43(2):109–42.
9. Michel T. NO way to relax: the complexities of coupling nitric oxide synthase pathways in the heart. Circulation 2010;121(4):519–28.
10. Schultz HD. Nitric oxide regulation of autonomic function in heart failure. Curr Heart Fail Rep 2009; 6(2):71–80.
11. Prabhu SD. Nitric oxide protects against pathological ventricular remodeling: reconsideration of the role of NO in the failing heart. Circ Res 2004; 94(9):1155–7.
12. Barouch LA, Harrison RW, Skaf MW, et al. Nitric oxide regulates the heart by spatial confinement of nitric oxide synthase. Nature 2002;416(6878): 337–9.
13. Hare JM. Spatial confinement of isoforms of cardiac nitric-oxide synthase: unraveling the complexities of nitric oxide's cardiobiology. Lancet 2004;363(9418):1338–9.
14. Cai H, Harrison DG. Endothelial dysfunction in cardiovascular diseases: the role of oxidant stress. Circ Res 2000;87:840–4.
15. Damy T, Ratajczak P, Robidel E, et al. Up-regulation of cardiac nitric oxide synthase 1-derived nitric oxide after myocardial infarction in senescent rats. FASEB J 2003;17(13):1934–6.
16. Damy T, Ratajczak P, Shah AM, et al. Increased neuronal nitric oxide synthase-derived NO production in the failing human heart. Lancet 2004; 363(9418):1365–7.
17. Drexler H, Hayoz D, Munzel T, et al. Endothelial function in chronic congestive heart failure. Am J Cardiol 1992;69(19):1596–601.
18. Heusch G, Boengler K, Schulz R. Cardioprotection: nitric oxide, protein kinases, and mitochondria. Circulation 2008;118(19):1915–9.
19. Mohri M, Egashira K, Tagawa T, et al. Basal release of nitric oxide is decreased in the coronary circulation in patients with heart failure. Hypertension 1997;30(1Pt1):50–6.
20. Recchia FA, McConnell PI, Bernstein RD, et al. Reduced nitric oxide production and altered myocardial metabolism during the decompensation of pacing-induced heart failure in the conscious dog. Circ Res 1998;83(10):969–79.

21. Ruiz-Hurtado G, Delgado C. Nitric oxide pathway in hypertrophied heart: new therapeutic uses of nitric oxide donors. J Hypertens 2010;28(Suppl 1): S56–61.

22. Saraiva RM, Hare JM. Nitric oxide signaling in the cardiovascular system: implications for heart failure. Curr Opin Cardiol 2006;21(3):221–8.

23. Umar S, van der Laarse A. Nitric oxide and nitric oxide synthase isoforms in the normal, hypertrophic, and failing heart. Mol Cell Biochem 2010; 333(1–2):191–201.

24. Winlaw D, Smythe G, Keogh AM, et al. Increased nitric oxide production in heart failure. Lancet 1994;344:373–4.

25. Zimmet JM, Hare JM. Nitroso-redox interactions in the cardiovascular system. Circulation 2006; 114(14):1531–44.

26. Gonzalez DR, Treuer A, Sun QA, et al. S-Nitrosylation of cardiac ion channels. J Cardiovasc Pharmacol 2009;54(3):188–95.

27. Hess DT, Foster MW, Stamler JS. Assays for S-nitrosothiols and S-nitrosylated proteins and mechanistic insights into cardioprotection. Circulation 2009;120(3):190–3.

28. Foster MW, Hess DT, Stamler JS. Protein S-nitrosylation in health and disease: a current perspective. Trends Mol Med 2009;15(9):391–404.

29. Lima B, Forrester MT, Hess DT, et al. S-nitrosylation in cardiovascular signaling. Circ Res 2010;106:633.

30. Gryglewski R, Palmer RM, Moncada S. Superoxide anion is involved in the breakdown of endothelium-derived vascular relaxing factor. Nature 1986;320: 454–6.

31. Guzik TJ, West NE, Black E, et al. Vascular superoxide production by NAD(P)H oxidase: association with endothelial dysfunction and clinical risk factors. Circ Res 2000;86(9):E85–90.

32. López Farré A, Casado S. Heart failure, redox alterations, and endothelial dysfunction. Hypertension 2001;38(6):1400–5.

33. Nediani C, Raimondi L, Borchi E, et al. Nitric oxide/reactive oxygen species generation and nitroso/redox imbalance in heart failure: from molecular mechanisms to therapeutic implications. Antioxid Redox Signal 2011;14(2):289–331.

34. Heymes C, Bendall JK, Ratajczak P, et al. Increased myocardial NADPH oxidase activity in human heart failure. J Am Coll Cardiol 2003;41(12):2164–71.

35. Keith M, Geranmayegan A, Sole MJ, et al. Increased oxidative stress in patients with congestive heart failure. J Am Coll Cardiol 1998;31(6):1352–6.

36. Kubo SH, Rector TS, Bank AJ, et al. Endothelium-dependent vasodilation is attenuated in patients with heart failure. Circulation 1991;84(4):1589–96.

37. Münzel T, Harrison DG. Increased superoxide in heart failure a biochemical baroreflex gone awry. Circulation 1999;100:216–8.

38. Sharma R, Davidoff MN. Oxidative stress and endothelial dysfunction in heart failure. Congest Heart Fail 2002;8(3):165–72.

39. Shizukuda Y, Buttrick PM. Oxygen free radicals and heart failure: new insight into an old question. Am J Physiol Lung Cell Mol Physiol 2002;283(2): L237–8.

40. Smith CJ, Sun D, Hoegler C, et al. Reduced gene expression of vascular endothelial NO synthase and cyclooxygenase-1 in heart failure. Circ Res 1996;78(1):58–64.

41. Takimoto E, Kass DA. Role of oxidative stress in cardiac hypertrophy and remodeling. Hypertension 2007;49(2):241–8.

42. Trachtenberg BH, Hare JM. Biomarkers of oxidative stress in heart failure. Heart Fail Clin 2009; 5(4):561–77.

43. Wang J, Seyedi N, Xu XB, et al. Defective endothelium mediated control of coronary circulation in conscious dogs after heart failure. Am J Physiol 1994;266:H670–80.

44. Diaz-Velez C, Garcia-Castineiras S, Mendoza-Ramos E, et al. Increased malondialdehyde peripheral blood of patients with congestive heart failure. Am Heart J 1996;131(1):146–52.

45. Belch J, Bridges AB, Scott N, et al. Oxygen free radicals and congestive heart failure. Br Heart J 1991;65:245–8.

46. Janssens S, Pokreisz P, Schoonjans L, et al. Cardiomyocyte-specific overexpression of nitric oxide synthase 3 improves left ventricular performance and reduces compensatory hypertrophy after myocardial infarction. Circ Res 2004;94(9): 1256–62.

47. Scherrer-Crosbie M, Ullrich R, Bloch KD, et al. Endothelial nitric oxide synthase limits left ventricular remodeling after myocardial infarction in mice. Circulation 2001;104(11):1286–91.

48. Takimoto E, Champion HC, Li M, et al. Oxidant stress from nitric oxide synthase-3 uncoupling stimulates cardiac pathologic remodeling from chronic pressure load. J Clin Invest 2005;115(5):1221–31.

49. Rohde D, Ritterhoff J, Voelkers M, et al. S100A1: a multifaceted therapeutic target in cardiovascular disease. J Cardiovasc Transl Res 2010;3(5):525–37.

50. Fraccarollo D, Widder JD, Galuppo P, et al. Improvement in left ventricular remodeling by the endothelial nitric oxide synthase enhancer AVE9488 after experimental myocardial infarction. Circulation 2008;118(8):818–27.

51. Ignarro L, Napoli C, Loscalzo J. Nitric oxide donors and cardiovascular agents modulating the bioactivity of nitric oxide. Circ Res 2002;90:21–8.

52. Chen Z, Zhang J, Stamler JS. Identification of the enzymatic mechanism of nitroglycerin bioactivation. Proc Natl Acad Sci U S A 2002;99(12): 8306–11.

53. Ignarro LJ, Lippton H, Edwards JC, et al. Mechanism of vascular smooth muscle relaxation by organic nitrates, nitrites, nitroprusside and nitric oxide: evidence for the involvement of S-nitrosothiols as active intermediates. J Pharmacol Exp Ther 1981;218(3):739–49.

54. Daiber A, Wenzel P, Oelze M, et al. New insights into bioactivation of organic nitrates, nitrate tolerance and cross-tolerance. Clin Res Cardiol 2008; 97(1):12–20.

55. Ignarro LJ. After 130 years, the molecular mechanism of action of nitroglycerin is revealed. Proc Natl Acad Sci U S A 2002;99(12):7816–7.

56. den Uil CA, Caliskan K, Lagrand WK, et al. Dose-dependent benefit of nitroglycerin on microcirculation of patients with severe heart failure. Intensive Care Med 2009;35(11):1893–9.

57. Sydow K, Daiber A, Oelze M, et al. Central role of mitochondrial aldehyde dehydrogenase and reactive oxygen species in nitroglycerin tolerance and cross-tolerance. J Clin Invest 2004;113(3): 482–9.

58. Parker JD. Nitrate tolerance, oxidative stress, and mitochondrial function: another worrisome chapter on the effects of organic nitrates. J Clin Invest 2004;113(3):352–4.

59. Gori T, Dragoni S, Di Stolfo G, et al. Tolerance to nitroglycerin-induced preconditioning of the endothelium: a human in vivo study. Am J Physiol Heart Circ Physiol 2010;298(2):H340–5.

60. Thomas GR, DiFabio JM, Gori T, et al. Once daily therapy with isosorbide-5-mononitrate causes endothelial dysfunction in humans: evidence of a free-radical-mediated mechanism. J Am Coll Cardiol 2007;49(12):1289–95.

61. Dragoni S, Gori T, Lisi M, et al. Pentaerythrityltetranitrate and nitroglycerin, but not isosorbide mononitrate, prevent endothelial dysfunction induced by ischemia and reperfusion. Arterioscler Thromb Vasc Biol 2007;27(9):1955–9.

62. Daiber A, Wenzel P, Oelze M, et al. Mitochondrial aldehyde dehydrogenase (ALDH-2)—maker of and marker for nitrate tolerance in response to nitroglycerin treatment. Chem Biol Interact 2009; 178(1–3):40–7.

63. Elkayam U. Nitrates in the treatment of congestive heart failure. Am J Cardiol 1996;77:41C–51C.

64. Elkayam U, Bitar F. Effects of nitrates and hydralazine in heart failure: clinical evidence before the African American Heart Failure Trial. Am J Cardiol 2005;96(7B):37i–43i.

65. Packer M, Lee WH, Kessler PD, et al. Prevention and reversal of nitrate tolerance in patients with congestive heart failure. N Engl J Med 1987; 317(13):799–804.

66. Unger P, Berkenboom G, Fontaine J. Interaction between hydralazine and nitrosovasodilators in vascular smooth muscle. J Cardiovasc Pharmacol 1993;21:478–83.

67. Daiber A, Oelze M, Coldewey M, et al. Hydralazine is a powerful inhibitor of peroxynitrite formation as a possible explanation for its beneficial effects on prognosis in patients with congestive heart failure. Biochem Biophys Res Commun 2005;338(4):1865–74.

68. Münzel T, Kurz S, Rajagopalan S, et al. Hydralazine prevents nitroglycerin tolerance by inhibiting activation of a membrane-bound NADH oxidase. A new action for an old drug. J Clin Invest 1996; 98(6):1465.

69. Leiro JM, Álvarez E, Arranz JA, et al. Antioxidant activity and inhibitory effects of hydralazine on inducible NOS/COX-2 gene and protein expression in rat peritoneal macrophages. Int Immunopharmacol 2004;4(2):163–77.

70. Bauer JA, Fung HL. Concurrent hydralazine administration prevents nitroglycerin-induced hemodynamic tolerance in experimental heart failure. Circulation 1991;84(1):35–9.

71. Gogia H, Mehra A, Parikh S, et al. Prevention of tolerance to hemodynamic effects of nitrates with concomitant use of hydralazine in patients with chronic heart failure. J Am Coll Cardiol 1995; 26(7):1575–80.

72. Cohn JN, Archibald DG, Ziesche S, et al. Effect of vasodilator therapy on mortality in chronic congestive heart failure. N Engl J Med 1986;314: 1547–52.

73. Cohn JN, Johnson G, Ziesche S, et al. A comparison of enalapril with hydralazine-isosorbide dinitrate in the treatment of chronic congestive heart failure. N Engl J Med 1991;325:303–10.

74. The Seventh Report of the Joint National Committee on Prevention, Detection, Evaluation, and Treatment of High Blood Pressure—complete report. NIH Publication No. 03-5231. Washington, DC: National Heart, Lung, and Blood Institute; 2003.

75. Exner D, Dries DL, Domanski MJ, et al. Lesser response to angiotensin-converting-enzyme inhibitor therapy in black as compared with white patients with left ventricular dysfunction. N Engl J Med 2001;344(18):1351–7.

76. Carson P, Ziesche S, Johnson G, et al. Racial differences in response to therapy for heart failure: analysis of the vasodilator-heart failure trials. J Card Fail 1999;5(3):178–87.

77. Franciosa JA, Taylor AL, Cohn JN, et al. African-American Heart Failure Trial (A-HeFT): rationale, design, and methodology. J Card Fail 2002;8: 128–35.

78. Taylor AL, Ziesche S, Yancy C, et al. Combination of isosorbide dinitrate and hydralazine in blacks with heart failure. N Engl J Med 2004;351(20): 2049–57.

79. Taylor AL, Lindenfeld J, Ziesche S, et al. Outcomes by gender in the African-American Heart Failure Trial. J Am Coll Cardiol 2006;48:2263–7.

80. Ghali JK, Tam SW, Sabolinski ML, et al. Exploring the potential synergistic action of spironolactone on nitric oxide-enhancing therapy: insights from the African American Heart Failure Trial. J Card Fail 2008;4:718–23.

81. Farguharson CA, Struthers AD. Spironolactone increases nitric oxide bioactivity, improves endothelial vasodilator dysfunction, and suppresses vascular angiotensin I/angiotensin II conversion in patients with chronic heart failure. Circulation 2000;101(6):594–7.

82. Cohn JN, Tam SW, Anand IS, et al. Isosorbide dinitrate and hydralazine in a fixed-dose combination produces further regression of left ventricular remodeling in a well-treated black population with heart failure: results from A-HeFT. J Card Fail 2007;13(5):331–9.

83. Mitchell J, Tam W, Trivedi K, et al. Atrial fibrillation and mortality in African American patients with heart failure: results from the African American Heart Failure Trial (A-HeFT). Am Heart J 2011; 162(1):154–9.

84. Anand I, Tam SW, Rector T, et al. Influence of blood pressure on the effectiveness of isosorbide dinitrate and hydralazine combination in the African-American Heart Failure Trial. J Am Coll Cardiol 2007;49:32–9.

85. Cohn JN, Ziesche S, Smith R, et al. Effect of the calcium antagonist felodipine as supplementary vasodilator therapy in patients with chronic heart failure treated with enalapril: V-HeFT III. Vasodilator-Heart Failure Trial (V-HeFT) Study Group. Circulation 1997;96:856–63.

86. Packer M, O'Connor CM, Ghali JK, et al. Effect of amlodipine on morbidity and mortality in severe chronic heart failure. Prospective Randomized Amlodipine Survival Evaluation Study Group. N Engl J Med 1996;335:1107–14.

87. Boerrigter G, Burnett JC Jr. Soluble guanylate cyclase: not a dull enzyme. Circulation 2009; 119(21):2752–4.

88. Ignarro LJ, Adams JB, Horwitz PM, et al. Activation of soluble guanylate cyclase by NO-hemoproteins involves NO-heme exchange. Comparison of heme-containing and heme-deficient enzyme forms. J Biol Chem 1986;261(11):4997–5002.

89. Priviero FB, Webb RC. Heme-dependent and independent soluble guanylate cyclase activators and vasodilation. J Cardiovasc Pharmacol 2010;56(3): 229–33.

90. Ritchie RH, Irvine JC, Rosenkranz AC, et al. Exploiting cGMP-based therapies for the prevention of left ventricular hypertrophy: NO* and beyond. Pharmacol Ther 2009;124(3):279–300.

91. Stasch JP, Pacher P, Evgenov OV. Soluble guanylate cyclase as an emerging therapeutic target in cardiopulmonary disease. Circulation 2011; 123(20):2263–73.

92. Ko FN, Wu CC, Kuo SC, et al. YC-1, a novel activator of platelet guanylate cyclase. Blood 1994; 84(12):4226–33.

93. Stasch JP, Becker EM, Alonso-Alija C, et al. NO-independent regulatory site on soluble guanylate cyclase. Nature 2001;410(6825):212–5.

94. Boerrigter G, Costello-Boerrigter LC, Cataliotti A, et al. Cardiorenal and humoral properties of a novel direct soluble guanylate cyclase stimulator BAY 41-2272 in experimental congestive heart failure. Circulation 2003;107(5):686–9.

95. Boerrigter G, Costello-Boerrigter LC, Cataliotti A, et al. Targeting heme-oxidized soluble guanylate cyclase in experimental heart failure. Hypertension 2007;49(5):1128–33.

96. Stasch JP, Schmidt P, Alonso-Alija C, et al. NO- and haem-independent activation of soluble guanylyl cyclase: molecular basis and cardiovascular implications of a new pharmacological principle. Br J Pharmacol 2002;136(5):773–83.

97. Mitrovic V, Hernandez AF, Meyer M, et al. Role of guanylate cyclase modulators in decompensated heart failure. Heart Fail Rev 2009;14(4):309–19.

98. Boerrigter G, Burnett JC Jr. Nitric oxide-independent stimulation of soluble guanylate cyclase with BAY 41-2272 in cardiovascular disease. Cardiovasc Drug Rev 2007;25(1):30–45.

99. Hingorany S, Frishman WH. Soluble guanylate cyclase activation with cinaciguat: a new approach to the treatment of decompensated heart failure. Cardiol Rev 2011;19(1):23–9.

100. Korkmaz S, Radovits T, Barnucz E, et al. Pharmacological activation of soluble guanylate cyclase protects the heart against ischemic injury. Circulation 2009;120(8):677–86.

101. Evgenov OV, Pacher P, Schmidt PM, et al. NO-independent stimulators and activators of soluble guanylate cyclase: discovery and therapeutic potential. Nat Rev Drug Discov 2006;5(9):755–68.

102. Ghofrani HA, Voswinckel R, Gall H. Riociguat for pulmonary hypertension. Future Cardiol 2010; 6(2):155–66.

103. Belik J. Riociguat, an oral soluble guanylate cyclase stimulator for the treatment of pulmonary hypertension. Curr Opin Investig Drugs 2009;10(9):971–9.

104. Schäfer A, Fraccarollo D, Werner L, et al. Guanylyl cyclase activator cinaciguat improves vascular function and reduces platelet activation in heart failure. Pharmacol Res 2010;62(5):432–8.

105. Lapp H, Mitrovic V, Franz N, et al. Cinaciguat (BAY 58-2667) improves cardiopulmonary hemodynamics in patients with acute decompensated heart failure. Circulation 2009;119(21):2781–8.

106. Mueck W, Frey R. Population pharmacokinetics and pharmacodynamics of cinaciguat, a soluble guanylate cyclase activator, in patients with acute decompensated heart failure. Clin Pharmacokinet 2010;49(2):119–29.

107. Grimminger F, Weimann G, Frey R, et al. First acute haemodynamic study of soluble guanylate cyclase stimulator riociguat in pulmonary hypertension. Eur Respir J 2009;33(4):785–92.

108. Kass DA, Takimoto E, Nagayama T, et al. Phosphodiesterase regulation of nitric oxide signaling. Cardiovasc Res 2007;75(2):303–14.

109. Kass DA, Champion HC, Beavo JA. Phosphodiesterase type 5: expanding roles in cardiovascular regulation. Circ Res 2007;101(11):1084–95.

110. Fischmeister R, Castro LR, Abi-Gerges A, et al. Compartmentation of cyclic nucleotide signaling in the heart: the role of cyclic nucleotide phosphodiesterases. Circ Res 2006;99(8):816–28.

111. Galiè N, Ghofrani HA, Torbicki A, et al. Sildenafil use in pulmonary Arterial Hypertension (SUPER) Study Group. Sildenafil citrate therapy for pulmonary arterial hypertension. N Engl J Med 2005; 353(20):2148–57.

112. Galiè N, Brundage BH, Ghofrani HA, et al. Pulmonary Arterial Hypertension and Response to Tadalafil (PHIRST) Study Group. Tadalafil therapy for pulmonary arterial hypertension. Circulation 2009; 119(22):2894–903.

113. Lu Z, Xu X, Hu X, et al. Oxidative stress regulates left ventricular PDE5 expression in the failing heart. Circulation 2010;121(13):1474–83.

114. Nagendran J, Archer SL, Soliman D, et al. Phosphodiesterase type 5 is highly expressed in the hypertrophied human right ventricle, and acute inhibition of phosphodiesterase type 5 improves contractility. Circulation 2007;116(3):238–48.

115. Pokreisz P, Vandenwijngaert S, Bito V, et al. Ventricular phosphodiesterase-5 expression is increased in patients with advanced heart failure and contributes to adverse ventricular remodeling after myocardial infarction in mice. Circulation 2009; 119(3):408–16.

116. Takimoto E, Champion HC, Li M, et al. Chronic inhibition of cyclic GMP phosphodiesterase 5A prevents and reverses cardiac hypertrophy. Nat Med 2005;11(2):214–22.

117. Nagayama T, Hsu S, Zhang M, et al. Sildenafil stops progressive chamber, cellular, and molecular remodeling and improves calcium handling and function in hearts with pre-existing advanced hypertrophy caused by pressure overload. J Am Coll Cardiol 2009;53(2):207–15.

118. Lewis GD, Lachmann J, Camuso J, et al. Sildenafil improves exercise hemodynamics and oxygen uptake in patients with systolic heart failure. Circulation 2007;115(1):59–66.

119. Lindman BR, Chakinala MM. Modulating the nitric oxide-cyclic GMP pathway in the pressure-overloaded left ventricle and group II pulmonary hypertension. Int J Clin Pract Suppl 2010;64(168): 15–22.

120. Lewis GD, Shah R, Shahzad K, et al. Sildenafil improves exercise capacity and quality of life in patients with systolic heart failure and secondary pulmonary hypertension. Circulation 2007;116(14): 1555–62.

121. Lewis GD, Semigran MJ. Type 5 phosphodiesterase inhibition in heart failure and pulmonary hypertension. Curr Heart Fail Rep 2004;1(4):183–9.

122. Behling A, Rohde LE, Colombo FC, et al. Effects of 5′-phosphodiesterase four-week long inhibition with sildenafil in patients with chronic heart failure: a double-blind, placebo-controlled clinical trial. J Card Fail 2008;14(3):189–97.

123. Guazzi M, Samaja M, Arena R, et al. Long-term use of sildenafil in the therapeutic management of heart failure. J Am Coll Cardiol 2007;50(22): 2136–44.

124. Guazzi M, Vicenzi M, Arena R, et al. PDE5 inhibition with sildenafil improves left ventricular diastolic function, cardiac geometry, and clinical status in patients with stable systolic heart failure: results of a 1-year, prospective, randomized, placebo-controlled study. Circ Heart Fail 2011; 4(1):8–17.

Stage B Heart Failure: Rationale for Screening

John J. Atherton, MBBS, PhD, FRACP, FCSANZ[a,b],*

KEYWORDS

- Diagnosis • Heart failure • Screening
- Ventricular dysfunction • Asymptomatic

Heart failure imposes an increasing burden on limited health care resources in developed and emerging economies. Its overall prevalence continues to rise and it remains the most common reason for hospital admission in the elderly.[1,2] Yet, like the tip of an iceberg, these epidemiologic descriptors provide an incomplete picture of the actual burden of heart failure. Clinicians have focused on the clinical syndrome of heart failure in symptomatic patients largely because this subset is easier to define from hospital coding systems and generally leads the patient to seek medical attention. However, as emphasized by the American College of Cardiology Foundation/ American Heart Association (ACCF/AHA) heart failure classification, attention needs to shift to an earlier stage of the disease spectrum.[3] This approach has been applied in other areas, most notably in early cancer detection programs where high-risk individuals are screened to identify presymptomatic disease.[4] However, there are a number of issues that need to be considered before embarking on such a strategy in heart failure.

First, one must define the current burden of suffering imposed by heart failure and whether this burden is adequately addressed. Then, it must be established whether those individuals at increased risk of developing symptomatic heart failure in the future can be identified and whether treating these high-risk individuals will lead to better clinical outcomes compared with waiting for patients to develop symptoms before deciding who and when to treat. Finally, presuming that these high-risk individuals can be safely and reliably detected, it needs to be determined whether introducing a screening strategy will be clinically effective and cost effective.

WHAT IS THE BURDEN OF SUFFERING ASSOCIATED WITH HEART FAILURE?

A middle-aged adult has a 20% to 30% lifetime risk of developing symptomatic heart failure.[5,6] After a patient develops symptomatic heart failure, their outlook is generally poor with a median survival of 3 to 5 years and comparable expected life-years lost as many common cancers.[5,7–12] Although there are a number of treatments that have been shown to improve outcomes in patients with heart failure associated with left ventricular (LV) systolic dysfunction (LVSD),[3,13,14] given that these treatments are applied fairly late in the disease trajectory, their overall impact on heart failure survival in epidemiologic studies has been modest.[7–10,12]

There has been minimal progress in heart failure prevention such that incident rates remain little changed in community-based studies.[1,7,9,10,12] This coupled with modest improvements in

Conflicts of interest: The author has nothing to disclose.
[a] Department of Cardiology, Royal Brisbane and Women's Hospital, Butterfield Street, Herston, Brisbane, Queensland, Australia 4029
[b] University of Queensland School of Medicine, c/o Department of Cardiology, Royal Brisbane and Women's Hospital, Butterfield Street, Herston, Brisbane, Queensland, Australia 4029
* Corresponding author. Department of Cardiology, Royal Brisbane and Women's Hospital, Butterfield Street, Herston, Brisbane, Queensland, Australia 4029.
E-mail address: john_atherton@health.qld.gov.au

Heart Failure Clin 8 (2012) 273–283
doi:10.1016/j.hfc.2011.11.003
1551-7136/12/$ – see front matter © 2012 Elsevier Inc. All rights reserved

survival explain why age-adjusted prevalence continues to rise and heart failure remains a common reason for hospitalization in the elderly, with the latter comprising the dominant economic burden imposed by heart failure.[1,2,15] Akin to only chipping away at the exposed tip of an iceberg, an isolated focus on diagnosing and treating symptomatic heart failure will have limited impact on population morbidity and mortality as incident cases of symptomatic heart failure continue to surface from the submerged presymptomatic burden of disease. The focus needs to shift to an earlier stage in the disease spectrum to identify and potentially treat high-risk individuals before the development of symptomatic heart failure.

WHICH INDIVIDUALS ARE AT RISK OF DEVELOPING SYMPTOMATIC HEART FAILURE?

Longitudinal studies have identified a number of clinical risk factors and antecedents for the subsequent development of symptomatic heart failure including hypertension, low high-density lipoprotein cholesterol, diabetes mellitus, smoking, physical inactivity, less education, atrial fibrillation, atherosclerotic vascular disease, chronic kidney disease, obesity, strain pattern on the 12-lead electrocardiogram (ECG), increased LV mass, LV diastolic dysfunction, left atrial dilatation, LVSD, valvular heart disease, mitral annular calcification, aortic calcification, and aortic root dilatation.[16–31] The ACCF/AHA staging classification highlights the presymptomatic phase of heart failure, which includes various heart failure risk factors (stage A) and asymptomatic structural heart disease (stage B) followed by the development of symptomatic heart failure (stages C and D).[3] Applying this staging classification to a population-based, cross-sectional sample of residents aged 45 years and older, 22% were stage A, 34% were stage B, 12% were stage C, and 0.2% were stage D, thereby highlighting the hidden burden of presymptomatic heart failure.[32]

Although the structural changes that comprise stage B heart failure are relatively broad, LVSD has received most attention. Depending on the age of the population studied and the cut-off chosen to define LVSD, its prevalence in predominantly middle-aged and elderly adults varies between 2% and 8%, with higher rates reported in men and the elderly.[33–42] Approximately half of these subjects have no prior or current history of symptomatic heart failure (**Table 1**). Furthermore, most individuals with asymptomatic LVSD in the community have either preexisting vascular disease or ACCF/AHA stage A heart failure risk

factors.[34,41] In the Framingham cohort, the prevalence of previous hypertension, myocardial infarction, and diabetes was greater in subjects with (65%, 49%, and 19%) compared with those without (43%, 2%, and 8%) asymptomatic LVSD, respectively.[41] Indeed, LVSD prevalence rates have been reported to be as high as 10% to 30% in subjects with symptomatic vascular disease, hypertension, or diabetes, which could allow a targeted screening strategy.[33,34,38–40,43]

WHAT IS THE RISK ASSOCIATED WITH STAGE B HEART FAILURE?

In a population-based sample of middle-aged and elderly subjects, the 5-year survival of individuals with stage B heart failure was 96%.[32] This included a broad range of structural abnormalities including LV diastolic dysfunction (60%); LV enlargement (34%); echocardiographic LV hypertrophy (24%); LVSD (10%); previous myocardial infarction (8%); regional wall motion abnormalities (7%); moderate or severe valvular heart disease (5%); and LV hypertrophy on the ECG (2%). There was a fivefold increase in mortality risk associated with the transition from stages B to C heart failure, highlighting the need for early detection strategies to identify subjects before the development of symptoms.

LVSD in young adults has a strong independent association with the development of incident symptomatic heart failure with a lead-time of approximately 10 years.[29] Middle-aged and elderly subjects with asymptomatic LVSD are at particularly high risk of major cardiovascular events in the medium-term including symptomatic heart failure and death.[39,41,44–46] In the Framingham cohort, 26% of subjects with asymptomatic LVSD developed symptomatic heart failure during the next 5 years, nearly a fivefold increased risk compared with subjects with normal LV function.[41] This risk persisted even when individuals with prior myocardial infarction were excluded. Their median survival was 7.1 years and after adjusting for age, sex, and various clinical covariates, they had a 60% higher mortality (**Fig. 1**). Almost two-thirds of the deaths were cardiovascular and 43% of the coronary artery disease deaths occurred suddenly. Importantly, over half of the deaths occurred before the development of symptomatic heart failure. The risks were even higher in subjects with asymptomatic moderate-to-severe LVSD who had an 8.5-fold increased risk of developing heart failure and a median survival of 5.4 years.[41] In the Studies of Left Ventricular Dysfunction (SOLVD)-Prevention trial, which enrolled predominantly middle-aged individuals with an LV ejection

Table 1
Prevalence of LVSD in community surveys involving more than 1000 subjects

Study	Sample Size	Age Range (years)	Mean Age (years)	LVSD Definition	Prevalence (%)	Proportion Symptom-Free (%)
McDonagh et al[34] (Scotland)	1467	25–74	50	EF ≤30%	2.9	48
				EF ≤35%	7.7	77
Schunkert et al[35] (Germany)	1566	25–75	50	EF <48%	2.7	42
Mosterd et al[36] (Netherlands)	2267	55–95	66	FS ≤25%	3.7	60
Davies et al[37] (England)	3960	≥45	61	EF <40%	1.8	47
				EF <50%	5.3	61
Devereaux et al[38] (USA)	3184	45–74	60	EF <40%	2.9	72
				EF <54%	14	90
Gottdiener et al[39] (USA)	5532	≥65	73	EF <45%	3.5	69
Redfield et al[40] (USA)	2042	≥45	63	EF ≤40%	2	47
				EF ≤50%	6	76
Wang et al[41] (USA)[a]	4257	40–95	61	EF ≤50%	3	
				EF <40%	1.2	
Abhayaratna et al[42] (Australia)	1275	60–86	69	EF ≤40%	2.1	22
				EF ≤50%	5.9	59
Bibbins-Domingo et al[29] (USA)	4230	23–35	30	EF <40%	0.4	

Abbreviations: EF, ejection fraction; FS, fractional shortening.
   [a] Subjects with a preexisting diagnosis of heart failure were excluded.
   Modified from Atherton JJ. Screening for left ventricular systolic dysfunction: is imaging a solution? JACC Cardiovasc Imaging 2010;3:423; with permission.

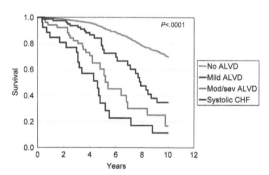

Fig. 1. Kaplan-Meier curves for survival of participants from the Framingham Study. Referent group consists of subjects with normal LV systolic function (ejection fraction [EF] >50%) and no history of congestive heart failure. Mild ALVD, mild asymptomatic LV systolic dysfunction (EF 40%–50%); Mod/Sev ALVD, moderate-to-severe asymptomatic LV systolic dysfunction (EF <40%); Systolic CHF, congestive heart failure with EF ≤50%. (*From* Wang TJ, Evans JC, Benjamin EJ, et al. Natural history of asymptomatic left ventricular systolic dysfunction in the community. Circulation 2003;108:979; with permission.)

fraction (LVEF) of 35% or less who were not receiving drug treatment for heart failure, approximately one in four subjects who were randomized to receive placebo died or were hospitalized with heart failure over 37-months follow-up, with more than 90% of the deaths being cardiovascular.[46] Therefore, waiting for individuals with asymptomatic LVSD to develop symptomatic heart failure represents a potential missed opportunity to modify the heart failure disease trajectory.

WILL EARLY DETECTION AND TREATMENT OF STAGE B HEART FAILURE IMPROVE CLINICAL OUTCOMES?

Although many structural cardiac abnormalities have been identified as heart failure antecedents, it is less well established that treating these asymptomatic high-risk individuals (in addition to the treatment they would usually receive based on their clinical risk factors) leads to better outcomes. For example, individuals with LV hypertrophy are at increased risk of cardiovascular events[30,47,48] and lowering blood pressure decreases the risk of death and incident heart failure in patients with hypertension; however, this benefit occurs whether or not LV hypertrophy is present.[49] LV hypertrophy may be a more appropriate treatment target than an arbitrary blood pressure level; however, the treatment efficacy studies to date have not been designed to address this.[50] In a small, placebo-controlled, randomized trial of asymptomatic, high-risk prehypertensive or controlled hypertensive subjects with functional or structural cardiovascular alterations on noninvasive testing, valsartan increased vascular elasticity and reduced blood pressure at 6 months, which translated to a reduction in LV mass at 12 months.[51] However, larger studies are required to assess the effect of this disease marker–targeted approach on long-term clinical outcomes.[52]

It remains unclear how one should treat individuals with isolated LV diastolic dysfunction in the presence or absence of heart failure symptoms with uniformly disappointing results in the treatment efficacy studies evaluating the management of heart failure associated with preserved LV systolic function.[53–55] However, neurohormonal antagonists promote reverse LV remodeling, improve symptoms, reduce heart failure hospitalization, and decrease mortality in patients with heart failure caused by LVSD.[3,13,14] Given that neurohormonal activation occurs in asymptomatic LVSD and is associated with an adverse prognosis, one should consider commencing these agents before the development of symptoms.[56]

Numerous large, randomized, placebo-controlled trials have established the benefit of inhibiting the renin–angiotensin system in symptomatic[57–59] and asymptomatic[46,58–60] LVSD. The strongest evidence in support of this approach comes from the SOLVD-Prevention trial in which individuals with asymptomatic moderate-to-severe LVSD were randomized to receive either enalapril or placebo.[46] The angiotensin-converting enzyme (ACE) inhibitor reduced the combined endpoint of death or heart failure hospitalization. The mortality reduction was highly significant in a subsequent 11-year follow-up analysis with a 9-month extension in life expectancy, despite most subjects probably receiving almost 9 years of open-label ACE inhibitor therapy after the study was completed (**Fig. 2**).[61] A strategy of commencing ACE inhibitors in subjects with asymptomatic LVSD was associated with improved long-term clinical outcomes compared with waiting for these subjects to develop symptomatic heart failure before deciding who and when to treat.

Given the undisputed benefit of β-blockers in patients with mild, moderate, and severe

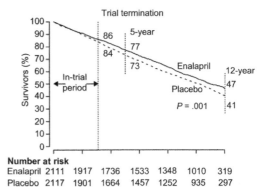

Fig. 2. Survival curves for the enalapril and placebo groups in the SOLVD-Prevention trial. Numbers beside the curves denote the percentage of survivors at termination, 5 years, and 12 years after randomization, calculated Kaplan-Meier method. (*From* Jong P, Yusuf S, Rousseau MF, et al. Effect of enalapril on 12-year survival and life expectancy in patients with left ventricular systolic dysfunction: a follow-up study. Lancet 2003;361:1845; with permission.)

symptomatic systolic heart failure[3,13,14] and the limitations of relying on a self-reported history to determine functional status, it seems reasonable to extend this indication to "asymptomatic" LVSD. Observational analyses in the SOLVD-Prevention and Survival and Ventricular Enlargement trials provide further support; subjects who received open-label β-blockers at baseline had a significantly lower risk of death and worsening heart failure in addition to the benefit seen with ACE inhibitor therapy.[62,63] An observational study in elderly patients with asymptomatic LVSD after myocardial infarction demonstrated significantly greater reductions in new coronary events and the development of heart failure with the combined use of ACE inhibitors and β-blockers compared with using either of these agents alone.[64] Furthermore, in the Carvedilol Post-Infarct Survival Control in LV Dysfunction trial in which almost all subjects were receiving ACE inhibitor therapy at baseline, there was a 23% lower mortality in the patients randomized to receive carvedilol, with similar benefit reported in a subgroup analysis of patients with no evidence of heart failure.[65,66] A recent placebo-controlled study provides mechanistic support with a significant reduction in LV end-systolic volume and increase in LVEF in subjects with asymptomatic LVSD randomized to receive 200 mg of extended-release metoprolol succinate.[67]

A large proportion of deaths in subjects with asymptomatic LVSD are sudden, most likely related to ventricular arrhythmia.[41] The Multicenter

Automatic Defibrillator Implantation Trial II evaluated the use of implantable cardioverter defibrillator therapy in patients with previous myocardial infarction and an LVEF of 30% or less.[68] A reduction in all-cause mortality was observed with a similar and significant benefit seen in patients with no symptoms of heart failure, suggesting this therapy may be considered in patients with a history of myocardial infarction associated with severe asymptomatic LVSD that persists despite ACE inhibitor and β-blocker therapy (**Table 2**).

Middle-aged men with coronary artery disease formed most subjects enrolled in the LVSD treatment efficacy studies. One may question whether it is reasonable to extrapolate these findings to a broader population. However, the consistent demonstration of benefit and the absence of significant heterogeneity with treatment effects being largely independent of age, sex, and etiology of LVSD supports their generalizability.[61,69,70] This is supported by the ACCF/AHA and European Society of Cardiology guidelines, which both recommend that individuals with asymptomatic LVSD should be treated with an ACE inhibitor regardless of whether or not they have had a previous myocardial infarct (class I recommendation).[3,13] Both guidelines also give a class I recommendation for the use of β-blockers to treat asymptomatic LVSD after myocardial infarction and the ACCF/AHA guidelines go further to recommend their use even without a history of previous myocardial infarction (see **Table 2**).

HOW SHOULD ONE EVALUATE A SCREENING STRATEGY?

Diagnostic tests generally have no direct effect on patient outcomes, but may do so indirectly by influencing the therapeutic pathway. With this in mind, Fineberg and colleagues[71] proposed more than three decades ago that a hierarchic approach with tiered levels of efficacy should be taken when evaluating diagnostic technologies. This model has subsequently been extended by others and involves evaluating the technical capabilities of a test (efficacy level 1); the diagnostic accuracy (efficacy level 2); the effect on the clinician's diagnostic thinking (efficacy level 3); the impact on the therapeutic plan (efficacy level 4); the effect on patient outcomes (efficacy level 5); and a consideration of the societal costs and benefits (efficacy level 6).[72,73] The final level is determined by all the lower levels of efficacy, the prevalence of disease in the target population where the test is applied, and local costs and reimbursement processes.

Ideally, to assess the effect of early detection of stage B heart failure on clinical outcomes, one would randomize subjects to either undergo a screening strategy to detect asymptomatic structural heart disease or to continue usual care (**Fig. 3**A).[74] Subjects with structural heart disease would then be treated whether they were detected systematically in the group randomized to undergo screening or fortuitously in the group randomized to continue with usual care. The outcomes of both groups would then be compared on an "intention to screen" basis providing direct evidence of the clinical effectiveness of screening for stage B heart failure. This approach allows one to balance the benefits of early disease detection and management with the potential risks associated with diagnostic procedures including the identification of false-positives and nontarget findings. Although this is generally regarded as the highest level of evidence being least prone to systematic bias, it is rarely performed for a variety of reasons including cost, ethical issues, and feasibility.

Table 2 ACCF/AHA and ESC Guidelines for treating asymptomatic LVSD (Recommendation; Level of Evidence)		
	ACCF/AHA Guidelines 2009[3]	**ESC Guidelines 2005[13]**
ACE I	(I; A)	(I; A)
Angiotensin receptor blockers	Post-MI and intolerant of ACE I (I; B) No prior MI and intolerant of ACE I (IIa; C)	Post-MI (I; A)
β-Blockers	Recent or remote MI (I; A) No prior MI (I; C)	Post-MI (I; B)
Implantable cardioverter defibrillator	≥40 days post-MI and LVEF ≤30% on optimal medical therapy (IIa; B) Nonischemic cardiomyopathy and LVEF ≤30% on optimal medical therapy (IIb; C)	

Abbreviations: ACE I, angiotensin-converting enzyme inhibitor; ESC, European Society of Cardiology; MI, myocardial infarction.

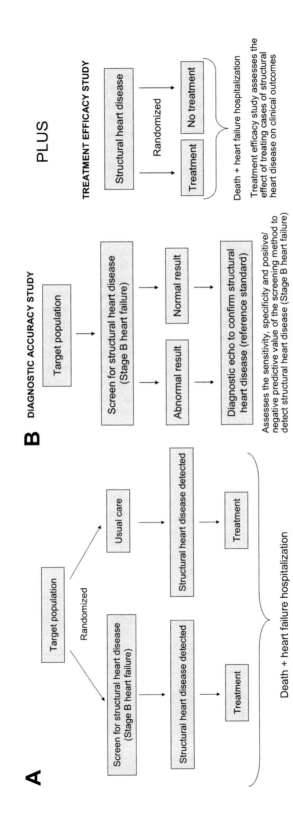

Fig. 3. Direct trial-based evidence (*A*) versus indirect linked evidence of diagnostic accuracy and treatment efficacy (*B*) to determine clinical effectiveness. (*Adapted from* Lord SJ, Irwig L, Simes RJ. When is measuring sensitivity and specificity sufficient to evaluate a diagnostic test, and when do we need randomized trials? Ann Intern Med 2006;144:851; with permission.)

Alternatively, if there is high-level evidence that treating subjects with structural heart disease leads to better clinical outcomes, one may infer the clinical effectiveness of a screening strategy that safely and reliably detects structural heart disease in a specified target population provided the cases detected represent the same spectrum of disease as the subjects enrolled in the treatment efficacy studies or the treatment effect is maintained across the disease spectrum (**Fig. 3**B).[74]

THE CASE FOR SCREENING FOR ASYMPTOMATIC LVSD

Despite recent advances in management, heart failure continues to impose a substantial clinical and financial burden on society. Numerous structural heart failure antecedents have been identified including asymptomatic LVSD, which contributes to loss of healthy life-years even before the development of symptoms,[41] with a strong body of evidence that treating these individuals leads to better outcomes.[46,58,59,61–68] Echocardiography is generally regarded as the gold standard for identifying LVSD; however, its limited availability and cost and the overall low prevalence of LVSD in the general community mandate the use of other methods to initially screen subjects. These methods include the use of clinical risk scores; the ECG; biomarkers, such as B-type natriuretic peptide; and hand-held echocardiography.[75–80]

Given that LVSD (usually determined by echocardiography or radionuclide ventriculography) has been used as a reference standard in diagnostic testing studies and as an inclusion criterion in the treatment efficacy studies, we can reasonably link the two approaches to infer clinical effectiveness.[81] If it is known that treating subjects with asymptomatic LVSD leads to better outcomes, then a screening strategy that safely and reliably detects asymptomatic LVSD should do the same. The consistent benefit seen in the treatment efficacy studies especially for ACE inhibitors across the spectrum of disease including patients with hypertension, vascular disease, asymptomatic LVSD, post-infarct LVSD, and systolic heart failure provides further support for using a linked evidence approach.[46,49,57,58,60,82–84] Furthermore, because most subjects in the community with undiagnosed asymptomatic LVSD are not taking ACE inhibitors,[85] one would expect that a strategy aimed at identifying these individuals and prescribing ACE inhibitors would lead to better outcomes. The question is therefore not whether one should treat asymptomatic LVSD, but whether doing so in the context of a screening program is clinically effective and cost effective.

In asymptomatic populations, a screening strategy with high specificity and positive predictive value will be favored to minimize the false-positive rate and subsequent unnecessary downstream investigations. This along with disease prevalence will be the dominant drivers of cost-effectiveness. A decision analytic model linking the treatment efficacy evidence for using ACE inhibitors in the SOLVD-Prevention study[46] with diagnostic accuracy evidence for using a B-type natriuretic peptide–based screening strategy followed by echocardiography in the Framingham population[76] concluded that screening for asymptomatic LVSD was cost effective provided its prevalence was at least 1% in the target population (**Fig. 4**).[86] The

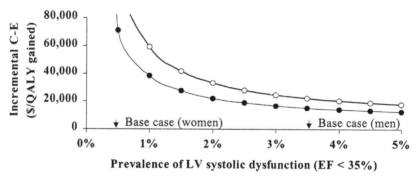

Fig. 4. Impact of prevalence of low EF on the cost-effectiveness (C–E) of screening for men and women using B-type natriuretic peptide (BNP) followed by echocardiography in those with a positive test. The cost-effectiveness ratio drops below $100,000 per quality-adjusted life-year (QALY) gained at a prevalence over 0.5% and drops below $50,000 at a prevalence over 1%. For any given prevalence of disease the cost-effectiveness ratio is lower for women because the accuracy of BNP is slightly greater for women than men. *Open circles*, men (BNP vs no screen); *closed circles*, women (BNP vs no screen). (*From* Heidenreich PA, Gubens MA, Fonarow GC, et al. Cost-effectiveness of screening with B-type natriuretic peptide to identify patients with reduced left ventricular ejection fraction. J Am Coll Cardiol 2004;43:1023; with permission.)

prevalence threshold clearly depends on reimbursement structures in different countries; however, in sensitivity analyses, screening and treatment costs had only a minor impact on the incremental cost-effectiveness ratio.[86]

Clinical effectiveness and cost effectiveness will be further enhanced by targeting populations with an increased prevalence of LVSD, such as patients with ischemic heart disease, diabetes mellitus, peripheral vascular disease, and cerebrovascular disease.[43,87]

SUMMARY

To adequately address the burden imposed by heart failure, a combined approach to prevention, early detection, and management is required. The ACCF/AHA heart failure classification appropriately draws attention to stages A and B heart failure with specific treatment recommendations being made in the guidelines. Failure to adequately consider this presymptomatic pool of subjects largely accounts for the continuing burden of incident cases of symptomatic heart failure. This article reviews the rationale for the early detection and management of stage B heart failure with specific reference to asymptomatic LVSD as a potentially modifiable heart failure antecedent. Provided one can safely and reliably detect these individuals, a strong case can be made for screening given the evidence from treatment efficacy studies that clinicians can improve patient outcomes.

REFERENCES

1. McCullough PA, Philbin EF, Spertus JA, et al. Confirmation of a heart failure epidemic: findings from the Resource Utilization Among Congestive Heart Failure (REACH) study. J Am Coll Cardiol 2002;39: 60–9.
2. Fang J, Mensah GA, Croft JB, et al. Heart failure-related hospitalization in the U.S., 1979 to 2004. J Am Coll Cardiol 2008;52:428–34.
3. Hunt SA, Abraham WT, Chin MH, et al. 2009 focused update incorporated into the ACC/AHA 2005 guidelines for the diagnosis and management of heart failure in adults. A report of the American College of Cardiology Foundation/American Heart Association Task Force on Practice Guidelines developed in collaboration with the International Society for Heart and Lung Transplantation. J Am Coll Cardiol 2009;53:e1–90.
4. Jacobsen SJ, Bergstralh EJ, Guess HA, et al. Predictive properties of serum-prostate-specific antigen testing in a community-based setting. Arch Intern Med 1996;156:2462–8.
5. Bleumink GS, Knetsch AM, Sturkenboom MC, et al. Quantifying the heart failure epidemic: prevalence, incidence rate, lifetime risk and prognosis of heart failure. The Rotterdam Study. Eur Heart J 2004;25:1614–9.
6. Lloyd-Jones DM, Larson MG, Leip EP, et al. Lifetime risk for developing congestive heart failure: the Framingham Heart Study. Circulation 2002;106: 3068–72.
7. Levy D, Kenchaiah S, Larson MG, et al. Long-term trends in the incidence of and survival with heart failure. N Engl J Med 2002;347:1397–402.
8. Owan TE, Hodge DO, Herges RM, et al. Trends in prevalence and outcome of heart failure with preserved ejection fraction. N Engl J Med 2006; 355:251–9.
9. Roger VL, Weston SA, Redfield MM, et al. Trends in heart failure incidence and survival in a community-based population. JAMA 2004;292:344–50.
10. Senni M, Tribouilloy CM, Rodeheffer RJ, et al. Congestive heart failure in the community: trends in incidence and survival in a 10-year period. Arch Intern Med 1999;159:29–34.
11. Stewart S, MacIntyre K, Hole DJ, et al. More "malignant" than cancer? Five-year survival following a first admission for heart failure. Eur J Heart Fail 2001;3: 315–22.
12. Gomez-Soto FM, Andrey JL, Garcia-Egido AA, et al. Incidence and mortality of heart failure: a community-based study. Int J Cardiol 2010;151(1):40–5.
13. Swedberg K, Cleland J, Dargie H, et al. Guidelines for the diagnosis and treatment of chronic heart failure: executive summary (update 2005). The Task Force for the Diagnosis and Treatment of Chronic Heart Failure of the European Society of Cardiology. Eur Heart J 2005;26:1115–40.
14. Krum H, Jelinek MV, Stewart S, et al. Guidelines for the prevention, detection and management of people with chronic heart failure in Australia 2006. Med J Aust 2006;185:549–57.
15. Stewart S, Jenkins A, Buchan S, et al. The current cost of heart failure to the National Health Service in the UK. Eur J Heart Fail 2002;4:361–71.
16. Gottdiener JS, Arnold AM, Aurigemma GP, et al. Predictors of congestive heart failure in the elderly: the Cardiovascular Health Study. J Am Coll Cardiol 2000;35:1628–37.
17. Aurigemma GP, Gottdiener JS, Shemanski L, et al. Predictive value of systolic and diastolic function for incident congestive heart failure in the elderly: the cardiovascular health study. J Am Coll Cardiol 2001;37:1042–8.
18. He J, Ogden LG, Bazzano LA, et al. Risk factors for congestive heart failure in US men and women: NHANES I epidemiologic follow-up study. Arch Intern Med 2001;161:996–1002.
19. Haider AW, Larson MG, Franklin SS, et al. Systolic blood pressure, diastolic blood pressure, and pulse

pressure as predictors of risk for congestive heart failure in the Framingham Heart Study. Ann Intern Med 2003;138:10–6.

20. Lam CS, Han L, Ha JW, et al. The mitral L wave: a marker of pseudonormal filling and predictor of heart failure in patients with left ventricular hypertrophy. J Am Soc Echocardiogr 2005;18: 336–41.

21. Barasch E, Gottdiener JS, Larsen EK, et al. Clinical significance of calcification of the fibrous skeleton of the heart and aortosclerosis in community dwelling elderly. The Cardiovascular Health Study (CHS). Am Heart J 2006;151:39–47.

22. Kizer JR, Bella JN, Palmieri V, et al. Left atrial diameter as an independent predictor of first clinical cardiovascular events in middle-aged and elderly adults: the Strong Heart Study (SHS). Am Heart J 2006;151:412–8.

23. Gardin JM, Arnold AM, Polak J, et al. Usefulness of aortic root dimension in persons ≥65 years of age in predicting heart failure, stroke, cardiovascular mortality, all-cause mortality and acute myocardial infarction (from the Cardiovascular Health Study). Am J Cardiol 2006;97:270–5.

24. Gottdiener JS, Kitzman DW, Aurigemma GP, et al. Left atrial volume, geometry, and function in systolic and diastolic heart failure of persons ≥65 years of age (the Cardiovascular Health Study). Am J Cardiol 2006;97:83–9.

25. Okin PM, Devereux RB, Nieminen MS, et al. Electrocardiographic strain pattern and prediction of new-onset congestive heart failure in hypertensive patients: the Losartan Intervention for Endpoint Reduction in Hypertension (LIFE) study. Circulation 2006;113:67–73.

26. Bibbins-Domingo K, Chertow GM, Fried LF, et al. Renal function and heart failure risk in older black and white individuals: the Health, Aging, and Body Composition Study. Arch Intern Med 2006;166: 1396–402.

27. Lee DS, Massaro JM, Wang TJ, et al. Antecedent blood pressure, body mass index, and the risk of incident heart failure in later life. Hypertension 2007;50:869–76.

28. de Simone G, Gottdiener JS, Chinali M, et al. Left ventricular mass predicts heart failure not related to previous myocardial infarction: the Cardiovascular Health Study. Eur Heart J 2008;29:741–7.

29. Bibbins-Domingo K, Pletcher MJ, Lin F, et al. Racial differences in incident heart failure among young adults. N Engl J Med 2009;360:1179–90.

30. Gardin JM, McClelland R, Kitzman D, et al. M-mode echocardiographic predictors of six- to seven-year incidence of coronary heart disease, stroke, congestive heart failure, and mortality in an elderly cohort (the Cardiovascular Health Study). Am J Cardiol 2001;87:1051–7.

31. Kalogeropoulos A, Georgiopoulou V, Kritchevsky SB, et al. Epidemiology of incident heart failure in a contemporary elderly cohort: the health, aging, and body composition study. Arch Intern Med 2009; 169:708–15.

32. Ammar KA, Jacobsen SJ, Mahoney DW, et al. Prevalence and prognostic significance of heart failure stages: application of the American College of Cardiology/American Heart Association heart failure staging criteria in the community. Circulation 2007; 115:1563–70.

33. Gardin JM, Siscovick D, Anton-Culver H, et al. Sex, age, and disease affect echocardiographic left ventricular mass and systolic function in the free-living elderly. The Cardiovascular Health Study. Circulation 1995;91:1739–48.

34. McDonagh TA, Morrison CE, Lawrence A, et al. Symptomatic and asymptomatic left-ventricular systolic dysfunction in an urban population. Lancet 1997;350:829–33.

35. Schunkert H, Broeckel U, Hense HW, et al. Left-ventricular dysfunction. Lancet 1998;351:372.

36. Mosterd A, Hoes AW, de Bruyne MC, et al. Prevalence of heart failure and left ventricular dysfunction in the general population. The Rotterdam Study. Eur Heart J 1999;20:447–55.

37. Davies M, Hobbs F, Davis R, et al. Prevalence of left-ventricular systolic dysfunction and heart failure in the Echocardiographic Heart of England Screening Study: a population based study. Lancet 2001;358: 439–44.

38. Devereux RB, Roman MJ, Paranicas M, et al. A population-based assessment of left ventricular systolic dysfunction in middle-aged and older adults: the Strong Heart Study. Am Heart J 2001; 141:439–46.

39. Gottdiener JS, McClelland RL, Marshall R, et al. Outcome of congestive heart failure in elderly persons: influence of left ventricular systolic function. The Cardiovascular Health Study. Ann Intern Med 2002;137:631–9.

40. Redfield MM, Jacobsen SJ, Burnett JC Jr, et al. Burden of systolic and diastolic ventricular dysfunction in the community: appreciating the scope of the heart failure epidemic. JAMA 2003;289:194–202.

41. Wang TJ, Evans JC, Benjamin EJ, et al. Natural history of asymptomatic left ventricular systolic dysfunction in the community. Circulation 2003; 108:977–82.

42. Abhayaratna WP, Smith WT, Becker NG, et al. Prevalence of heart failure and systolic ventricular dysfunction in older Australians: the Canberra Heart Study. Med J Aust 2006;184:1–154.

43. Kelly R, Struthers AD. Screening for left ventricular systolic dysfunction in patients with stroke, transient ischaemic attacks, and peripheral vascular disease. QJM 1999;92:295–7.

44. McDonagh TA, Cunningham AD, Morrison CE, et al. Left ventricular dysfunction, natriuretic peptides, and mortality in an urban population. Heart 2001;86:21–6.

45. Lauer MS, Evans JC, Levy D. Prognostic implications of subclinical left ventricular dilatation and systolic dysfunction in men free of overt cardiovascular disease (the Framingham Heart Study). Am J Cardiol 1992;70:1180–4.

46. Effect of enalapril on mortality and the development of heart failure in asymptomatic patients with reduced left ventricular ejection fractions. The SOLVD Investigators. N Engl J Med 1992;327: 685–91.

47. Verdecchia P, Schillaci G, Borgioni C, et al. Prognostic value of a new electrocardiographic method for diagnosis of left ventricular hypertrophy in essential hypertension. J Am Coll Cardiol 1998;31:383–90.

48. Levy D, Garrison RJ, Savage DD, et al. Prognostic implications of echocardiographically determined left ventricular mass in the Framingham Heart Study. N Engl J Med 1990;322:1561–6.

49. Turnbull F. Effects of different blood-pressure-lowering regimens on major cardiovascular events: results of prospectively-designed overviews of randomised trials. Lancet 2003;362:1527–35.

50. Devereux RB, Wachtell K, Gerdts E, et al. Prognostic significance of left ventricular mass change during treatment of hypertension. JAMA 2004;292:2350–6.

51. Duprez DA, Florea ND, Jones K, et al. Beneficial effects of valsartan in asymptomatic individuals with vascular or cardiac abnormalities: the DETECTIV Pilot Study. J Am Coll Cardiol 2007;50:835–9.

52. Cohn JN, Duprez DA. Time to foster a rational approach to preventing cardiovascular morbid events. J Am Coll Cardiol 2008;52:327–9.

53. Massie BM, Carson PE, McMurray JJ, et al. Irbesartan in patients with heart failure and preserved ejection fraction. N Engl J Med 2008;359:2456–67.

54. Yusuf S, Pfeffer MA, Swedberg K, et al. Effects of candesartan in patients with chronic heart failure and preserved left-ventricular ejection fraction: the CHARM-Preserved Trial. Lancet 2003;362:777–81.

55. Cleland JG, Tendera M, Adamus J, et al. The perindopril in elderly people with chronic heart failure (PEP-CHF) study. Eur Heart J 2006;27:2338–45.

56. Benedict CR, Shelton B, Johnstone DE, et al. Prognostic significance of plasma norepinephrine in patients with asymptomatic left ventricular dysfunction. SOLVD Investigators. Circulation 1996;94: 690–7.

57. Effect of enalapril on survival in patients with reduced left ventricular ejection fractions and congestive heart failure. The SOLVD Investigators. N Engl J Med 1991;325:293–302.

58. Kober L, Torp-Pedersen C, Carlsen JE, et al. A clinical trial of the angiotensin-converting-enzyme inhibitor trandolapril in patients with left ventricular dysfunction after myocardial infarction. Trandolapril Cardiac Evaluation (TRACE) Study Group. N Engl J Med 1995;333:1670–6.

59. Pfeffer MA, McMurray JJ, Velazquez EJ, et al. Valsartan, captopril, or both in myocardial infarction complicated by heart failure, left ventricular dysfunction, or both. N Engl J Med 2003;349: 1893–906.

60. Pfeffer MA, Braunwald E, Moye LA, et al. Effect of captopril on mortality and morbidity in patients with left ventricular dysfunction after myocardial infarction. Results of the Survival and Ventricular Enlargement Trial. The SAVE Investigators. N Engl J Med 1992;327:669–77.

61. Jong P, Yusuf S, Rousseau MF, et al. Effect of enalapril on 12-year survival and life expectancy in patients with left ventricular systolic dysfunction: a follow-up study. Lancet 2003;361:1843–8.

62. Vantrimpont P, Rouleau JL, Wun CC, et al. Additive beneficial effects of beta-blockers to angiotensin-converting enzyme inhibitors in the Survival and Ventricular Enlargement (SAVE) Study. SAVE Investigators. J Am Coll Cardiol 1997;29:229–36.

63. Exner DV, Dries DL, Waclawiw MA, et al. Beta-adrenergic blocking agent use and mortality in patients with asymptomatic and symptomatic left ventricular systolic dysfunction: a post hoc analysis of the studies of left ventricular dysfunction. J Am Coll Cardiol 1999;33:916–23.

64. Aronow WS, Ahn C, Kronzon I. Effect of beta blockers alone, of angiotensin-converting enzyme inhibitors alone, and of beta blockers plus angiotensin-converting enzyme inhibitors on new coronary events and on congestive heart failure in older persons with healed myocardial infarcts and asymptomatic left ventricular systolic dysfunction. Am J Cardiol 2001;88:1298–300.

65. Dargie HJ. Effect of carvedilol on outcome after myocardial infarction in patients with left-ventricular dysfunction: the CAPRICORN randomised trial. Lancet 2001;357:1385–90.

66. Goldberg LR, Jessup M. Stage B heart failure: management of asymptomatic left ventricular systolic dysfunction. Circulation 2006;113:2851–60.

67. Colucci WS, Kolias TJ, Adams KF, et al. Metoprolol reverses left ventricular remodeling in patients with asymptomatic systolic dysfunction: the REversal of VEntricular Remodeling with Toprol-XL (REVERT) trial. Circulation 2007;116:49–56.

68. Moss AJ, Zareba W, Hall WJ, et al. Prophylactic implantation of a defibrillator in patients with myocardial infarction and reduced ejection fraction. N Engl J Med 2002;346:877–83.

69. Flather MD, Yusuf S, Kober L, et al. Long-term ACE-inhibitor therapy in patients with heart failure or left-ventricular dysfunction: a systematic overview of data from individual patients. ACE-Inhibitor

Myocardial Infarction Collaborative Group. Lancet 2000;355:1575–81.

70. Packer M, Coats AJ, Fowler MB, et al. Effect of carvedilol on survival in severe chronic heart failure. N Engl J Med 2001;344:1651–8.

71. Fineberg HV, Bauman R, Sosman M. Computerized cranial tomography. Effect on diagnostic and therapeutic plans. JAMA 1977;238:224–7.

72. Fryback DG, Thornbury JR. The efficacy of diagnostic imaging. Med Decis Making 1991;11:88–94.

73. Gazelle GS, McMahon PM, Siebert U, et al. Cost-effectiveness analysis in the assessment of diagnostic imaging technologies. Radiology 2005;235:361–70.

74. Lord SJ, Irwig L, Simes RJ. When is measuring sensitivity and specificity sufficient to evaluate a diagnostic test, and when do we need randomized trials? Ann Intern Med 2006;144:850–5.

75. Kannel WB, D'Agostino RB, Silbershatz H, et al. Profile for estimating risk of heart failure. Arch Intern Med 1999;159:1197–204.

76. Vasan RS, Benjamin EJ, Larson MG, et al. Plasma natriuretic peptides for community screening for left ventricular hypertrophy and systolic dysfunction: the Framingham Heart Study. JAMA 2002;288:1252–9.

77. Davenport C, Cheng EY, Kwok YT, et al. Assessing the diagnostic test accuracy of natriuretic peptides and ECG in the diagnosis of left ventricular systolic dysfunction: a systematic review and meta-analysis. Br J Gen Pract 2006;56:48–56.

78. Ewald B, Ewald D, Thakkinstian A, et al. Meta-analysis of B type natriuretic peptide and N-terminal pro B natriuretic peptide in the diagnosis of clinical heart failure and population screening for left ventricular systolic dysfunction. Intern Med J 2008;38:101–13.

79. Redfield MM, Rodeheffer RJ, Jacobsen SJ, et al. Plasma brain natriuretic peptide to detect preclinical ventricular systolic or diastolic dysfunction: a community-based study. Circulation 2004;109:3176–81.

80. Galasko GI, Lahiri A, Senior R. Portable echocardiography: an innovative tool in screening for cardiac abnormalities in the community. Eur J Echocardiogr 2003;4:119–27.

81. Atherton JJ. Screening for left ventricular systolic dysfunction: is imaging a solution? JACC Cardiovasc Imaging 2010;3:421–8.

82. Yusuf S, Sleight P, Pogue J, et al. Effects of an angiotensin-converting-enzyme inhibitor, ramipril, on cardiovascular events in high-risk patients. The Heart Outcomes Prevention Evaluation Study Investigators. N Engl J Med 2000;342:145–53.

83. Fox KM. Efficacy of perindopril in reduction of cardiovascular events among patients with stable coronary artery disease: randomised, double-blind, placebo-controlled, multicentre trial (the EUROPA study). Lancet 2003;362:782–8.

84. Cohn JN, Johnson G, Ziesche S, et al. A comparison of enalapril with hydralazine-isosorbide dinitrate in the treatment of chronic congestive heart failure. N Engl J Med 1991;325:303–10.

85. Ho SF, O'Mahony MS, Steward JA, et al. Left ventricular systolic dysfunction and atrial fibrillation in older people in the community: a need for screening? Age Ageing 2004;33:488–92.

86. Heidenreich PA, Gubens MA, Fonarow GC, et al. Cost-effectiveness of screening with B-type natriuretic peptide to identify patients with reduced left ventricular ejection fraction. J Am Coll Cardiol 2004;43:1019–26.

87. Galasko GI, Barnes SC, Collinson P, et al. What is the most cost-effective strategy to screen for left ventricular systolic dysfunction: natriuretic peptides, the electrocardiogram, hand-held echocardiography, traditional echocardiography, or their combination? Eur Heart J 2006;27:193–200.

Strategies to Screen for Stage B as a Heart Failure Prevention Intervention

Margaret M. Redfield, MD

KEYWORDS

- Heart failure • Screening • Population studies • Prevention

Screening for stage B heart failure (HF) is based on the concept that asymptomatic alterations in left ventricular (LV) structure or function (stage B HF) identify patients at increased risk for progression to overt (stage C) HF and that interventions in stage B HF prevent or substantially delay this progression and reduce the burden of HF in the population.

The approach to screening and intervention to prevent a condition is dictated by the prevalence and natural history of the condition and its susceptibility to therapeutic intervention. The natural history and therapeutics of HF are intimately linked to those of vascular disease and hypertension and, increasingly, to those of a host of noncardiovascular comorbidities that represent competing risks for morbidity and mortality in patients with or at risk for overt HF and contribute to the progression of HF.

The approach to screening for stage B HF is influenced by the scope of the definition of stage B HF. Stage B HF is broadly termed structural and functional cardiac abnormalities but has been narrowly defined as previous myocardial infarction (MI) with regional dysfunction or scar, LV hypertrophy (LVH), reduced ejection fraction (EF), or structural valve disease.[1] This definition is likely more dictated by limitations in the type of abnormalities that can be reliably measured with current technology rather than the current understanding of the structural and functional cardiovascular perturbations that cause HF progression (as addressed in sections A and B of this issue). Although most paradigms for detection of stage B HF focus on biomarkers and imaging tests to detect a single abnormality, a clinical HF risk score could serve as a surrogate marker for stage B HF by identifying patients with cumulative derangements in cardiac and vascular structure and function that may not be easily characterized by conventional imaging but predispose to HF progression. Thus, clinical HF risk scores can also be considered a screening test.

The approach to screening for stage B HF is also influenced by the scope of the target for prevention and the type of intervention being tested. HF is a clinical syndrome with 2 broad phenotypes of approximately equal prevalence in the community.[2,3] These phenotypes include HF with preserved or reduced EF. These 2 phenotypes share many common features, but there are important differences that seem (to date) to be associated with differential response to therapies.[4] A strategy testing interventions to prevent all HF may need screening only to establish increased risk of HF. Here, novel approaches to risk factor modification within a health care system or novel agents that ameliorate pathophysiologic features common to both forms of HF (myocyte hypertrophy, fibrosis, diastolic dysfunction, vascular dysfunction) or contributing comorbidities (renal dysfunction) could be tested.

PREVALENCE AND NATURAL HISTORY OF STAGE B HF AND IMPLICATIONS FOR SCREENING
Reduced EF

Asymptomatic LV systolic dysfunction (EF ≤50%) is estimated to be present in 3% to 6% of the adult

Cardiovascular Division, Mayo Clinic, 200 First Street, Southwest, Rochester, MN 55905, USA
E-mail address: redfield.margaret@mayo.edu

Heart Failure Clin 8 (2012) 285–296
doi:10.1016/j.hfc.2011.12.001
1551-7136/12/$ – see front matter © 2012 Elsevier Inc. All rights reserved.

population, with the majority (approximately 70%) of affected individuals being men and most (60%–70%) having mild reduction in EF (between 40% and 50%).[5–8] In the Olmsted County Heart Study, a cross-sectional echocardiographic survey of the general population older than 45 years, the prevalence of asymptomatic reduction in EF (≤50%) was much higher in the elderly (>65 years) with known coronary disease or hypertension (16.8%, men; 5.0%, women) than in the general population (7.9%, men; 2.2%, women).[5] In the Framingham Heart Study (FHS), the prevalence of asymptomatic EF of 50% or less increased dramatically with age in men (2.1% in those aged 40–59 years, 7.2% in those aged 60–69 years, 11.3% in those aged 70–79 years, and 14.3% in those aged ≥80 years) but was less than 1.0% in all but the oldest (≥80 years) women (1.9% with asymptomatic EF ≤50%).[6] Similarly, the Cardiovascular Health Study (CHS) enrolled noninstitutionalized persons older than 65 years and did not exclude those with prevalent coronary or cerebrovascular disease. In the CHS, the prevalence of reduced EF was 7.3%, with 68% being men and the majority (66%) having borderline reduction in EF (defined as 45%–55% in this study).

Data from randomized clinical trials enrolling patients with asymptomatic decrease in EF suggest that average annual HF incidence ranges from 5% to 20%, although these trials were heavily skewed toward younger patients with known coronary disease and more severe LV systolic dysfunction (entry criteria of EF <35%–40%).[9–11] In the community, data from the FHS confirm that persons with asymptomatic reduction in EF had an HF incidence of 5.8 per 100 person-years.[6] In the CHS, the HF incidence rate (median follow-up of 11.7 years) was 5.7 per 100 person-years in persons with asymptomatic reduction in EF, as compared with 2.4 per 100 person-years in those with normal EF.[8]

LVH

Electrocardiographic or echocardiographic evidence of LVH or echocardiographically defined concentric remodeling is common in patients with hypertension, particularly in the setting of renal dysfunction. Studies in untreated hypertensive patients suggest that the prevalence of LVH is 10% to 30% in those with mild-moderate hypertension and 50% to 60% in those with more severe hypertension.[12] The Olmsted County Heart study showed that in participants (>45 years of age) without HF but with a diagnosis of hypertension, concentric remodeling (21%), concentric hypertrophy (21%), and eccentric hypertrophy (19%)

were common.[13] Patients with concentric remodeling (without increased LV mass) as well as concentric and eccentric LVH are at increased risk for cardiovascular events.[12,14,15] Regression or prevention of development of echocardiographic or electrocardiographic LVH over time is associated with reduced adverse cardiovascular events, but convincing data indicating that LVH regression, above and beyond blood pressure control, prevents future HF events are lacking.[12,15] Although transition from concentric hypertrophy to systolic HF is common in several animal models of pressure overload, the frequency with which this happens in humans is unclear. Several recent studies suggest that although abnormal LV geometry is a risk factor for HF, progression from concentric LVH to dilated cardiomyopathy in the absence of an intercurrent MI is uncommon (<20%).[15]

LV Diastolic Dysfunction

Estimates of the prevalence of diastolic dysfunction vary by methods used to define it. The Olmsted County Heart Study showed that mild diastolic dysfunction (abnormal relaxation pattern) was common (17.9% of community participants older than 45 years) and increased in prevalence with age, whereas 6.7% had moderate or severe diastolic dysfunction (pseudonormal or restrictive pattern). Older (>65 years) patients with a diagnosis of hypertension or coronary disease had a much higher prevalence of mild (36%) or moderate or severe (16%) diastolic dysfunction. Diastolic dysfunction was independently associated with poorer outcomes in this study.[5] A follow-up of the Olmsted County study and a recent analysis from the FHS have reported that various diastolic function parameters are independent risk factors (adjusted hazard ratios in 1.3–1.6 range) for incident HF.[16,17] Although no therapy has been conclusively demonstrated to improve diastolic function independent of load or remodeling effects or to improve outcomes in overt HF with preserved EF, the presence of diastolic dysfunction does seem to identify patients at increased risk for HF.

Other Forms of Stage B HF

Current guidelines exist for screening of relatives of patients with idiopathic dilated or hypertrophic cardiomyopathy, as well as evaluation and follow-up of individuals during cardiotoxin exposure, with asymptomatic murmurs or documented structural valve disease.

Overall Burden of Stage B HF

The Olmsted County Heart Study showed that 23% of the population (older than 45 years) had stage B HF (prior MI, regional wall motion abnormality, LV dilatation, LVH, EF <50%, or structural valve disease) as defined by clinical, electrocardiographic, and Doppler echocardiographic assessment and that the prevalence of stage B HF increased to 34% if the definition of stage B HF included diastolic dysfunction and to 39% to 46% in participants older than 65 years (depending on definition of stage B HF).[18] Although there was a trend toward increased mortality for participants with stage B HF over 7 years of follow-up, this met statistical significance only in men; however, stage B HF is clearly associated with increased mortality when the definition is confined to those with reduced EF as outlined earlier. The Dallas Heart Study included a cardiac magnetic resonance (CMR) examination in 2339 participants (48% black) aged 30 to 65 years; defined stage B HF as the presence of LVH, reduced EF, or prior MI; and found that 12.5% of participants met the definition of stage B HF, with most subjects having LVH and 3% of participants having reduced EF.[19]

CRITERIA NEEDED TO JUSTIFY SCREENING PROGRAMS

Seven guidelines for determining whether a screening program is likely to be effective have been proposed.[20] Such guidelines are heavily considered in the approval of screening programs by organizations such as the US Preventative Services Task Force (USPSTF), which evaluate and make recommendations regarding screening services.[21] At present, few screening tests for cardiovascular disease have been endorsed by the USPSTF.

1. Has the effectiveness of the program been demonstrated in a randomized trial?

To date, no randomized trial has evaluated the impact of a strategy to screen for and treat stage B HF.

2. Are efficacious treatments available?

Randomized clinical trials in patients with asymptomatic LV systolic dysfunction (most with coronary disease or MI) and hypertension with LVH suggest several potentially efficacious and currently available therapies (renin-angiotensin-aldosterone system [RAAS] antagonists and β-blockers).[9] Extrapolation of data from previous large randomized clinical trials to estimate impact of community screening/treating is challenging because such cohorts differ in many important ways from unselected patients in the community who may be targeted in a screen-and-treat intervention. Patient characteristics, tolerance of and adherence to interventions, and effect size of interventions may differ in the unselected individual in the community.

3. Does the burden of suffering warrant screening?

The burden of HF in terms of morbidity, mortality, and health care resource use is well established and sufficient to justify a prevention intervention.[22] However, HF is by and large a disease of the elderly, with community-based studies showing that 80% of patients with incident HF are older than 65 years and 50% are older than 80 years.[23,24] In these individuals, cardiovascular and noncardiovascular comorbidities have important implications for any strategy designed to prevent HF. A community-based HF surveillance study has demonstrated that only a small fraction (<20%) of hospitalizations over the course of a patient's life after an HF diagnosis are for HF,[25] that health care use is concentrated in the last 6 months of life,[26] and that most patients with incident HF in the community die from coronary vascular disease and noncardiovascular comorbidities.[27] Thus, interventions designed to prevent or delay HF face the harsh reality of HF as a competing risk for other cardiovascular and noncardiovascular diseases that impair functional status, quality of life, and survival and contribute to health care resource use.

4. Is there a good screening test?

Several potential screening strategies exist, which are outlined later.

5. Does the program reach those who could benefit?

Clinical risk factor–based screening and biomarker-based screening are available uniformly. Such a strategy has distinct advantages because technology incorporated into an electronic medical record is modifying the concept of "screening," whereby a screening intervention can now be a continuous and passive process rather than a discrete active intervention. Imaging-based screening is somewhat less widely available.

6. Can the health system cope with the program?

Treatment of asymptomatic patients with an EF less than 40% with RAAS antagonists and β-blockers is already endorsed by guidelines.[22] Although treatment of patients with milder degrees of systolic dysfunction (EF, 40%–50%) has not been tested, extrapolation of the natural history of patients with this degree systolic dysfunction from numerous epidemiology studies suggest that if risk reduction was 10% to 30% with therapy, the number needed to treat to prevent HF in patients with mild EF reduction would be relatively small (17–52).[7] However, this finding may have relatively little impact on the burden of HF in the community as outlined later. The implications of treating patients with more common forms of stage B HF (abnormal geometry or diastolic dysfunction) or those at increased risk for HF but without standard criteria for stage B HF for the health care system are as yet undefined.

7. Do persons with positive screenings comply with advice and interventions?

Blood pressure screening is inexpensive, widely available, and promoted through many community-based education programs. Highly effective, well-tolerated, and (relatively) low-cost treatments are abundant, yet hypertension awareness, treatment, and control rates are only 71%, 61%, and 34%, respectively.[28] Similarly, the benefit of lipid-lowering therapy in at-risk individuals is well established, but adherence to long-term statin therapy is well below 50% in many studies.[29] Sobering recent data on patients with recent MI indicate poor (<50%) adherence even when medications are free.[30] The challenges to ensuring compliance with a therapy for any asymptomatic condition must be acknowledged.

POTENTIAL SCREENING STRATEGIES

Population-based studies that included baseline ("screening") echocardiography, risk scores and biomarkers, and longitudinal follow-up for HF incidence provide insight into the potential value of different screening strategies to reduce HF incidence and the burden of HF in the community.

Clinical Risk Factor–Based Screening for HF Risk

Two epidemiology studies have developed HF risk prediction scores (**Table 1**) that generally have only a moderate discriminative value for identifying whether or not an individual will develop overt HF (c index in the 0.7–0.8 range). The original FHS HF prediction score was developed in the late 1990s in individuals with hypertension, coronary heart disease, or valve disease and used simple clinical data available from the medical record. This risk score identified patients with incremental risk of future HF (see **Table 1**).[31] The Health Aging and Body Composition (ABC) study enrolled

3075 well-functioning community-dwelling elderly persons aged 70 to 79 years. No baseline echocardiography was performed, but data regarding incident HF were collected over time and a risk score (**Fig. 1**) predictive of incident HF at 5 years was derived from the data and compared with the FHS HF risk score. The ABC risk score was superior to the FHS score but still provided only moderate discrimination for incident HF (see **Table 1**).[32] Further refinements to clinical scoring systems may yield superior results because a subsequent analysis of a subset of the FHS cohort found that additional simple clinical variables predicted incident HF with a c index of 0.84 (Framingham Heart Study [FHS]-2, see **Table 1**).[33]

Although discrimination was only moderate with these risk scores, the calibration of the ABC score was excellent in the derivation study (the Health ABC study)[34] and, importantly, when applied to participants in the CHS (**Fig. 2**).[35] These 2 studies are particularly relevant because they enrolled older individuals who are at greatest risk for HF. Importantly, these studies also define the numbers of older individuals without prevalent HF who have low (<5%), average (5%–10%), high (10%–20%), and very high (>20%) risk of overt HF over 5 years and thus provide insight into the number of persons who would be suitable for an intervention to prevent HF based on an HF risk score. Further, the studies define the portion of patients with incident HF in the population who would have been identified by the HF score and thus the portion of the HF burden that could potentially be affected by a preventative strategy restricted to those identified as at higher risk (**Fig. 3** and **Table 2**). Findings in the ABC study and CHS were highly consistent and indicate that approximately 40% of older individuals have a risk more than 5% of HF over 5 years and that approximately 75% of HF events occur in these individuals. Thus, intervening with an HF prevention strategy in those at a risk of more than 5% of developing HF would limit the application of the intervention to 40% of the older population and offer the potential to affect 75% of future HF events. Intervening in those at more than 10% risk of developing HF would limit the application of the intervention to 20% of the older population and offer the potential to affect 50% of future HF events. Subsequent studies in the CHS cohort have also examined biomarkers, and thus the value of the ABC HF risk score, N-terminal pro-B-type natriuretic peptide (NT-proBNP), and screening echo as screening strategies can be compared in a robust cohort with extensive follow-up for incident HF (see later).

Table 1
Clinical risk scores for incident HF. Parameters included in the models, characteristics of the studies in which the models were developed, and predictive characteristics are shown

	FHS	ABC	FHS-2
Age	+	+	+
Prevalent Coronary Disease	+	+	−
LVH on Electrocardiography	+	+	−
Systolic Blood Pressure	+	+	+
Heart Rate	+	+	−
Smoking	−	+	−
Serum Albumin	−	+	+
Serum Creatinine	−	+	−
Fasting Blood Glucose	−	+	−
Diabetes Mellitus	+	−	+
Valve Disease	+	−	+
Body Mass Index	+ (women only)	−	+
Race	−	−	−
Gender	−	−	+
Antihypertensive Medication Use	−	−	+
N-Terminal Pro-B-Type Natriuretic Peptide	−	−	−
Total Cholesterol/High-Density Lipoprotein Cholesterol	…	…	+
MI	…	…	+
Cohort	15,267 p-examination	2853 persons	2754 persons
Men (%)	42	48	46
White (%)	Most	59	Most
Age Cohort (y)	45–94	70–79	59 ± 10
Definition of HF	Framingham	HF hsp	Framingham
Follow-Up (y)	38	7	9.4
HF Incidence (Cumulative) (%)	3.2	8.8	7.4
Predicted Variable	4-y risk of HF	5-y risk of HF	HF incidence
c Index	nr	0.784 (men); 0.750 (women)	0.84 (men & women)
c Index FHS Score in ABC Cohort	…	0.735 (men); 0.684 (women)	…

Data from Refs.[31–33]

Clinical Risk Factor–Based Screening for Stage B HF

The Dallas Heart Study examined the association of cardiac structure and function as assessed by CMR imaging within strata of HF risk as defined by the ABC HF risk score and showed that measures of LV mass (indexed to body size by several methods) and concentric remodeling increased across the HF risk strata, whereas eccentric remodeling (LV volume/body surface area) did not. EF did decline across the HF risk strata, but frank systolic dysfunction (EF less than the normal range for CMR) was uncommon (3%).[36] These data suggest that increased risk of HF is associated, on average, with structural heart disease. The HF prediction score may identify the cumulative subclinical alterations in cardiac and noncardiac structure and function that lead to future HF. This presents a less-well-defined discrete therapeutic target

Age	
Years	Points
≤71	-1
72-75	0
76-78	1
≥79	2

Heart Rate	
bpm	Points
≤50	-2
55-60	-1
65-70	0
75-80	1
85-90	2
≥95	3

Fasting Glucose	
mg/dl	Points
≤80	-1
85-125	0
130-170	1
175-220	2
225-265	3
≥270	5

Coronary Artery Disease	
Status	Points
No	0
Possible	2
Definite	5

Smoking	
Status	Points
Never	0
Past	1
Current	4

Creatinine	
mg/dl	Points
≤0.7	-2
0.8-0.9	-1
1.0-1.1	0
1.2-1.4	1
1.5-1.8	2
1.9-2.3	3
>2.3	6

LV Hypertrophy	
Status	Points
No	0
Yes	2

Albumin	
g/dl	Points
≥4.8	-3
4.5-4.7	-2
4.2-4.4	-1
3.9-4.1	0
3.6-3.8	1
3.3-3.5	2
≤3.2	3

Key:
Systolic BP to nearest 5mmHg
Heart Rate to nearest 5bpm
Albumin to nearest 0.1g/dl
Glucose to nearest 5mg/dl
Creatinin to nearest 0.1mg/dl

HF=Heart Failure

Systolic Blood Pressure	
mmHg	Points
≤90	-4
95-100	-3
105-115	-2
120-125	-1
130-140	0
145-150	1
155-165	2
170-175	3
180-190	4
195-200	5
>200	6

Health ABC HF Risk Score	HF Risk Group	5-yr HF Risk
≤2 points	Low	<5%
3-5 points	Average	5-10%
6-9 points	High	10-20%
≥10 points	Very High	>20%

Fig. 1. The Health ABC HF risk prediction score. (*Data from* Butler J, Kalogeropoulos A, Georgiopoulou V, et al. Incident heart failure prediction in the elderly: the health ABC heart failure score. Circ Heart Fail 2008;1(2): 125–33.)

but does not preclude the design of testable intervention strategies targeting those at highest risk for HF. Such strategies may include standard risk factor modification and monitoring with interventions to enhance compliance as well as novel agents that may address multiple pathways that lead to HF. An advantage of this approach is that the clinical risk score could be incorporated into electronic medical records, allowing continual passive screening to identify high-risk subjects with alerts for patients entering higher-risk strata to undergo an intervention.

Biomarker-Based Screening for HF Risk

Both the FHS and the ABC study have explored the ability of several biomarkers to enhance clinical scores for HF risk assessment. In the FHS, B-type natriuretic peptide (BNP) and the urinary albumin to creatinine ratio (but not C-reactive protein, plasminogen activator inhibitor 1, homocysteine, or aldosterone to renin ratio) increased the discrimination of a clinical HF prediction score modestly (increasing c index from 0.84 to 0.86).[33] However, 13% of subjects were appropriately reclassified as being in higher or lower different risk strata,

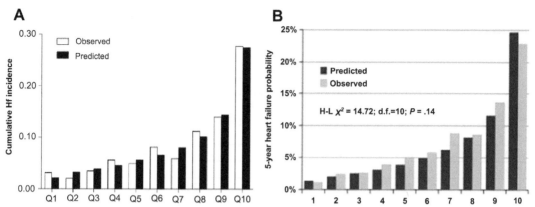

Fig. 2. Comparison of predicted and observed HF incidence across deciles of the Health ABC HF risk prediction score in the Health ABC study (*A*) and CHS (*B*). (*Data from* Butler J, Kalogeropoulos A, Georgiopoulou V, et al. Incident heart failure prediction in the elderly: the health ABC heart failure score. Circ Heart Fail 2008;1(2):125–33 [*A*]; and Kalogeropoulos A, Psaty BM, Vasan RS, et al. Validation of the health ABC heart failure model for incident heart failure risk prediction: the Cardiovascular Health Study. Circ Heart Fail 2010;3(4):495–502 [*B*].)

suggesting that biomarkers could better categorize patients into risk strata in which differential therapeutic approaches would be pursued. In the ABC study, the additive value of inflammatory markers (interleukin 6, tumor necrosis factor α, and C-reactive protein) to the ABC clinical risk score was assessed. Interleukin 6 provided modest but statistically significant additive

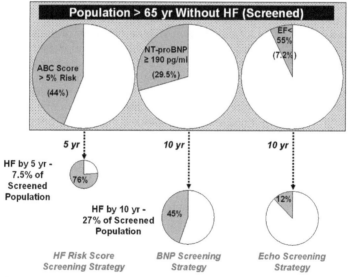

Fig. 3. The ABC HF risk score, *N*-terminal pro-B-type natriuretic peptide (NT-proBNP) levels, and echocardiography-based screening in the CHS cohort. The percentage of the cohort with a positive screening result, the percentage of the cohort who went on to develop incident HF, and the percentage of the patient who developed HF who would have been identified by the screening intervention are shown. The ABC HF risk score indicated higher (>5%) risk of HF at 5 years in 44% of the cohort and identified 76% of those who developed HF by 5 years. As the score was validated to predict 5-year risk of HF, only data on 5-year HF incidence were reported. An abnormal NT-proBNP level was present in 29.5% of the cohort and identified 45% of those who developed HF by 10 years. The baseline (screening) echocardiography identified reduced EF in 7.2% of the population, but a low EF on screening identified only 12% of those who developed HF by 10 years. (*Data from* Kalogeropoulos A, Psaty BM, Vasan RS, et al. Validation of the health ABC heart failure model for incident heart failure risk prediction: the Cardiovascular Health Study. Circ Heart Fail 2010;3(4):495–502; and deFilippi CR, Christenson RH, Kop WJ, et al. Left ventricular ejection fraction assessment in older adults: an adjunct to natriuretic peptide testing to identify risk of new-onset heart failure and cardiovascular death? J Am Coll Cardiol 2011;58(14):1497–506.)

Table 2
ABC HF risk prediction score in the ABC and CHS. Potential implications for targeting interventions and aing incident HF

Predicted 5-y HF Risk Category (%)	Health ABC Study			CHS		
	N	Observed 5-y HF Incidence (%)	Observed 5-y HF Events (n)	N	Observed 5-y HF Incidence (%)	Observed 5-y HF Events (n)
<5	1754	2.9	51	2985	3.2	95
5–10	618	5.7	35	1361	9.0	122
10–20	375	13.3	50	696	15.9	111
>20	106	36.8	39	293	24.6	72
Total	2853	—	175	5335	—	400

Data from Butler J, Kalogeropoulos A, Georgiopoulou V, et al. Incident heart failure prediction in the elderly: the health ABC heart failure score. Circ Heart Fail 2008;1(2):125–33; and Kalogeropoulos A, Psaty BM, Vasan RS, et al. Validation of the health ABC heart failure model for incident heart failure risk prediction: the Cardiovascular Health Study. Circ Heart Fail 2010;3(4):495–502.

discrimination (c index increased from 0.717 to 0.734) and improved the model fit as assessed by the Bayes information criterion, but reclassification was not assessed.[37] In the CHS, the additional value of NT-proBNP to clinical data for prediction of HF was assessed, but this analysis did not specifically use the ABC risk score. NT-proBNP value increased the c index for identification of participants who would develop HF from 0.667 (clinical data) to 0.719 ($P<.001$), but discrimination remained moderate at best. These studies suggest that HF risk stratification can be improved by biomarkers that might be useful if a prevention strategy was targeting those with increased HF risk rather than a specific abnormality in cardiac structure of function.

The data from the CHS cohort allow comparison of the ABC HF risk score, NT-proBNP value, and echocardiographic result to detect low EF as screening strategies for future HF.[35,38] The percentage of the cohort with a positive screening result, the percentage of the cohort who went on to develop incident HF, and the percentage of the patients who developed HF who would have been identified by the screening intervention are shown in **Fig. 3**. The ABC HF risk score indicated higher (>5%) risk of HF at 5 years in 44% of the cohort and identified 76% of those who developed HF by 5 years. As the score was validated to predict 5-year risk of HF, only data on 5-year HF incidence were reported. An abnormal NT-proBNP level was present in 29.5% of the cohort and identified 45% of those who developed HF by 10 years. The baseline (screening) echocardiography identified reduced EF in 7.2% of the population, but a low EF on screening identified only 12% of those who developed HF by 10 years.

Biomarker-Based Screening for Stage B HF

The Dallas Heart Study examined the ability of the ABC HF risk score, BNP, NT-proBNP, and the combination of BNP or NT-proBNP and clinical risk score to detect Stage B HF defined as LVH or reduced EF without an HF diagnosis.[19] The combination of a high clinical risk score and an elevated BNP or NT-proBNP had the best predictive characteristics for identifying Stage B HF (**Fig. 4**), but positive predictive values with partition values favoring specificity were still quite low and indicate that 70% of imaging studies obtained in response to screening would not identify LVH or systolic dysfunction. This study used CMR, and the use of a less-reproducible imaging technique, such as echocardiography, would likely result in even less robust results.

Both the FHS and the Olmsted County Heart Study have examined the potential utility of natriuretic peptides as a stand-alone screening intervention to detect asymptomatic LV systolic dysfunction or other types of stage B HF in the general population and simply defined (age, sex, known cardiovascular disease) high-risk groups.[39,40] Both these studies used statistical analyses that focused on defining the discriminatory value of natriuretic peptide assays for determining if an individual patient had various types of stage B HF. The implications for a BNP screening program to detect asymptomatic reduction in EF in the general population or

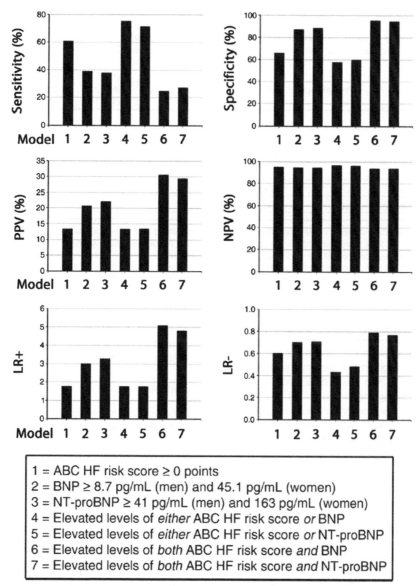

1 = ABC HF risk score ≥ 0 points
2 = BNP ≥ 8.7 pg/mL (men) and 45.1 pg/mL (women)
3 = NT-proBNP ≥ 41 pg/mL (men) and 163 pg/mL (women)
4 = Elevated levels of *either* ABC HF risk score *or* BNP
5 = Elevated levels of *either* ABC HF risk score *or* NT-proBNP
6 = Elevated levels of *both* ABC HF risk score *and* BNP
7 = Elevated levels of *both* ABC HF risk score *and* NT-proBNP

Fig. 4. The predictive characteristics of the Health ABC HF risk prediction score, natriuretic peptide assays, and their combination for detection of stage B HF. Data are from the Dallas Heart Study in which stage B HF was defined as previous MI, LR+, likelihood ratio of positive test; LR−, likelihood ratio of negative test; LVH, or reduced EF. NPV, negative predictive value; PPV, positive predictive value. (*Data from* Gupta S, Rohatgi A, Ayers CR, et al. Risk scores versus natriuretic peptides for identifying prevalent stage B heart failure. Am Heart J 2011;161(5):923–30, e922.)

a high-risk subset as defined in the Olmsted County Heart Study are shown in **Table 3**.[39] The predictive characteristics of BNP for detection of EF of 40% or less (c index of 0.82–0.92) were better than for detection of EF of 50% or less (c index of 0.51–0.74), but even focusing on detection of EF of 40% or less, the burden of imaging and yield on imaging would preclude a biomarker-only strategy from becoming widely accepted because most follow-up study results would be negative. A similar analysis with NT-proBNP in the same cohort was substantially identical.[41] Findings from the FHS were similar.[40] Although other investigators postulate that natriuretic peptides could be cost effective,[42] the low prevalence of systolic dysfunction provides a very high bar for a screening biomarker and the search continues for a biomarker or biomarker panel that could identify systolic dysfunction in an individual.

Table 3
Use of BNP assay to identify individuals with asymptomatic systolic dysfunction (EF ≤40%) in the general population and a higher-risk group studied in the Olmsted County Heart Study

	Prevalence (%)	Sensitivity (%)	Specificity (%)	Screened Needing Echo (%)	Echoes Negative (%)	Disease Missed (%)
Population	1.1	90	76	24	96	10
Age >65 y	2.0	80	72	29	94	20
Men	1.9	88	83	18	91	12
Women	0.3	67	87	13	98	33
High-Risk[a] Men	5.3	85	73	29	89	15
High-Risk[a] Women	0.6	50	82	18	99	50

Partition values based on optimal values identified on receiver operating characteristic analysis. Predictive characteristics for detection of EF ≤50% were markedly less robust. Findings with NT-proBNP were similar.[41]
    [a] High risk indicates age greater than 65 years with prevalent coronary disease or hypertension.
    Data from Redfield MM, Rodeheffer RJ, Jacobsen SJ, et al. Plasma brain natriuretic peptide to detect preclinical ventricular systolic or diastolic dysfunction: a community-based study. Circulation 2004;109(25):3176–81.

Imaging Screening to Detect Stage B HF

Although the prevalence of asymptomatic LV systolic dysfunction in the general adult population (3%–6%) is too low to advocate use of traditional imaging techniques as a primary screening modality, population studies have identified subsets with sufficient prevalence of systolic dysfunction (elderly men with prevalent cardiovascular disease in whom the prevalence of asymptomatic EF ≤50% was 17%) that may warrant a primary imaging strategy as is currently recommended for abdominal aortic aneurysm (1-time ultrasonography in men aged 65–75 years with a history of smoking).[21] Handheld echocardiography has the potential to greatly extend the availability of cardiac imaging.[43] However, training noncardiologists to use this technology is in its infancy, and sensitivity and specificity of noncardiologist-based echocardiography, particularly for milder reduction in EF, LVH, diastolic dysfunction, and valvular disease, is as yet undefined. Further, although the examination itself performed with a handheld machine by a minimally trained individual may be of lower cost, the cost of widespread purchase of these devices, training of individuals, and validation of performance indices would be considerable and not likely to be justified by the potential to detect reduced EF in asymptomatic persons alone. The potential for adverse consequences of false-positive screening as well as false-negative study results would need to be carefully considered. As demonstrated in **Fig. 3**, although the risk of HF is increased in persons with reduced EF and treatment with standard HF therapies may well reduce

the risk of future HF, focusing on this small segment of those at risk may not greatly reduce the burden of HF in the community.

SUMMARY

HF prevention is an indisputably laudable goal, albeit with undefined global public health impact in an increasingly elderly population with competing cardiovascular and noncardiovascular risks for morbidity and mortality. The understanding of cardiac and noncardiac structural and functional abnormalities that predispose to the diverse clinical HF syndrome is rapidly advancing, and novel approaches for prevention and treatment are needed. Successful approaches mandate not only identification of discrete therapeutic targets but also research into the developing sciences of health care delivery and behavioral modification. Targeting stage B HF represents one such potential strategy.

REFERENCES

1. Hunt SA, Baker DW, Chin MH, et al. ACC/AHA guidelines for the evaluation and management of chronic heart failure in the adult: a report of the American College of Cardiology/American Heart Association Task Force on Practice Guidelines (Committee to Revise the 1995 Guidelines for the Evaluation and Management of Heart Failure). Circulation 2001;104(24):2996–3007.
2. Owan TE, Hodge DO, Herges RM, et al. Trends in prevalence and outcome of heart failure with preserved ejection fraction. N Engl J Med 2006; 355(3):251–9.

3. Owan TE, Redfield MM. Epidemiology of diastolic heart failure. Prog Cardiovasc Dis 2005;47(5):320–32.

4. Borlaug BA, Redfield MM. Diastolic and systolic heart failure are distinct phenotypes within the heart failure spectrum. Circulation 2011;123(18):2006–14.

5. Redfield MM, Jacobsen SJ, Burnett JC Jr, et al. Burden of systolic and diastolic ventricular dysfunction in the community: appreciating the scope of the heart failure epidemic. JAMA 2003;289(2):194–202.

6. Wang TJ, Evans JC, Benjamin EJ, et al. Natural history of asymptomatic left ventricular systolic dysfunction in the community. Circulation 2003; 108(8):977–82.

7. Wang TJ, Levy D, Benjamin EJ, et al. The epidemiology of "asymptomatic" left ventricular systolic dysfunction: implications for screening. Ann Intern Med 2003;138:907–16.

8. Pandhi J, Gottdiener JS, Bartz TM, et al. Comparison of characteristics and outcomes of asymptomatic versus symptomatic left ventricular dysfunction in subjects 65 years old or older (from the Cardiovascular Health Study). Am J Cardiol 2011; 107(11):1667–74.

9. Goldberg LR, Jessup M. Stage B heart failure: management of asymptomatic left ventricular systolic dysfunction. Circulation 2006;113(24): 2851–60.

10. Pfeffer MA, Braunwald E, Moye LA, et al. Effect of captopril on mortality and morbidity in patients with left ventricular dysfunction after myocardial infarction. Results of the survival and ventricular enlargement trial. The SAVE Investigators. N Engl J Med 1992;327(10):669–77.

11. SOLVD-Investigators. Effect of enalapril on mortality and the development of heart failure in asymptomatic patients with reduced left ventricular ejections. N Engl J Med 1992;327:685–91.

12. Gradman AH, Alfayoumi F. From left ventricular hypertrophy to congestive heart failure: management of hypertensive heart disease. Prog Cardiovasc Dis 2006;48(5):326–41.

13. Lam CS, Roger VL, Rodeheffer RJ, et al. Cardiac structure and ventricular-vascular function in persons with heart failure and preserved ejection fraction from Olmsted County, Minnesota. Circulation 2007;115(15):1982–90.

14. Artham SM, Lavie CJ, Milani RV, et al. Clinical impact of left ventricular hypertrophy and implications for regression. Prog Cardiovasc Dis 2009;52(2):153–67.

15. Drazner MH. The progression of hypertensive heart disease. Circulation 2011;123(3):327–34.

16. Kane GC, Karon BL, Mahoney DW, et al. Progression of left ventricular diastolic dysfunction and risk of heart failure. JAMA 2011;306(8):856–63.

17. Lam CS, Lyass A, Kraigher-Krainer E, et al. Cardiac dysfunction and noncardiac dysfunction as precursors of heart failure with reduced and preserved ejection fraction in the community. Circulation 2011;124(1):24–30.

18. Ammar KA, Jacobsen SJ, Mahoney DW, et al. Prevalence and prognostic significance of heart failure stages: application of the American College of Cardiology/American Heart Association heart failure staging criteria in the community. Circulation 2007; 115(12):1563–70.

19. Gupta S, Rohatgi A, Ayers CR, et al. Risk scores versus natriuretic peptides for identifying prevalent stage B heart failure. Am Heart J 2011;161(5): 923–30, e922.

20. Cadman D, Chambers L, Feldman W, et al. Assessing the effectiveness of community screening programs. JAMA 1984;251(12):1580–5.

21. U.S. Preventative Services Task Force. Available at: http://www.uspreventiveservicestaskforce.org/index. html. Accessed November 29, 2011.

22. Hunt SA, Abraham WT, Chin MH, et al. 2009 focused update incorporated into the ACC/AHA 2005 guidelines for the diagnosis and management of heart failure in adults. A report of the American College of Cardiology Foundation/American Heart Association Task Force on practice guidelines developed in collaboration with the International Society for Heart and Lung Transplantation. J Am Coll Cardiol 2009;53(15):e1–90.

23. Roger VL, Weston SA, Redfield MM, et al. Trends in heart failure incidence and survival in a community-based population. JAMA 2004;292(3):344–50.

24. Senni M, Tribouilloy CM, Rodeheffer RJ, et al. Congestive heart failure in the community: a study of all incident cases in Olmsted County, Minnesota, in 1991. Circulation 1998;98(21):2282–9.

25. Dunlay SM, Redfield MM, Weston SA, et al. Hospitalizations after heart failure diagnosis a community perspective. J Am Coll Cardiol 2009;54(18):1695–702.

26. Dunlay SM, Shah ND, Shi Q, et al. Lifetime costs of medical care after heart failure diagnosis. Circ Cardiovasc Qual Outcomes 2011;4(1):68–75.

27. Henkel DM, Redfield MM, Weston SA, et al. Death in heart failure: a community perspective. Circ Heart Fail 2008;1(2):91–7.

28. Hajjar I, Kotchen TA. Trends in prevalence, awareness, treatment, and control of hypertension in the United States, 1988-2000. JAMA 2003;290(2): 199–206.

29. Bates TR, Connaughton VM, Watts GF. Non-adherence to statin therapy: a major challenge for preventive cardiology. Expert Opin Pharmacother 2009; 10(18):2973–85.

30. Choudhry NK, Avorn J, Glynn RJ, et al. Full coverage for preventive medications after myocardial infarction. N Engl J Med 2011;365(22):2088–97.

31. Kannel WB, D'Agostino RB, Silbershatz H, et al. Profile for estimating risk of heart failure. Arch Intern Med 1999;159(11):1197–204.

32. Butler J, Kalogeropoulos A, Georgiopoulou V, et al. Incident heart failure prediction in the elderly: the health ABC heart failure score. Circ Heart Fail 2008;1(2):125–33.

33. Velagaleti RS, Gona P, Larson MG, et al. Multimarker approach for the prediction of heart failure incidence in the community. Circulation 2010;122(17):1700–6.

34. Butter C, Gras D, Ritter P, et al. Comparative prospective randomized efficacy testing of different guiding catheters for coronary sinus cannulation in heart failure patients. J Interv Card Electrophysiol 2003;9(3):343–51.

35. Kalogeropoulos A, Psaty BM, Vasan RS, et al. Validation of the health ABC heart failure model for incident heart failure risk prediction: the Cardiovascular Health Study. Circ Heart Fail 2010;3(4):495–502.

36. Gupta S, Berry JD, Ayers CR, et al. Association of Health Aging and Body Composition (ABC) Heart Failure score with cardiac structural and functional abnormalities in young individuals. Am Heart J 2010;159(5):817–24.

37. Kalogeropoulos A, Georgiopoulou V, Psaty BM, et al. Inflammatory markers and incident heart failure risk in older adults: the Health ABC (Health, Aging, and Body Composition) study. J Am Coll Cardiol 2010; 55(19):2129–37.

38. deFilippi CR, Christenson RH, Kop WJ, et al. Left ventricular ejection fraction assessment in older adults: an adjunct to natriuretic peptide testing to identify risk of new-onset heart failure and cardiovascular death? J Am Coll Cardiol 2011;58(14): 1497–506.

39. Redfield MM, Rodeheffer RJ, Jacobsen SJ, et al. Plasma brain natriuretic peptide to detect preclinical ventricular systolic or diastolic dysfunction: a community-based study. Circulation 2004;109(25): 3176–81.

40. Vasan RS, Benjamin EJ, Larson MG, et al. Plasma natriuretic peptides for community screening for left ventricular hypertrophy and systolic dysfunction: the Framingham heart study. JAMA 2002;288(10): 1252–9.

41. Costello-Boerrigter LC, Boerrigter G, Redfield MM, et al. Amino-terminal pro-B-type natriuretic peptide and B-type natriuretic peptide in the general community: determinants and detection of left ventricular dysfunction. J Am Coll Cardiol 2006; 47(2):345–53.

42. Heidenreich PA, Gubens MA, Fonarow GC, et al. Cost-effectiveness of screening with B-type natriuretic peptide to identify patients with reduced left ventricular ejection fraction. J Am Coll Cardiol 2004;43(6):1019–26.

43. Atherton JJ. Screening for left ventricular systolic dysfunction: is imaging a solution? JACC Cardiovasc Imaging 2010;3(4):421–8.

Index

Note: Page numbers of article titles are in **boldface** type.

Heart Failure Clin 8 (2012) 297–300
doi:10.1016/S1551-7136(12)00012-8
1551-7136/12/$ – see front matter © 2012 Elsevier Inc. All rights reserved.

Moving?

Make sure your subscription moves with you!

To notify us of your new address, find your **Clinics Account Number** (located on your mailing label above your name), and contact customer service at:

Email: journalscustomerservice-usa@elsevier.com

800-654-2452 (subscribers in the U.S. & Canada)
314-447-8871 (subscribers outside of the U.S. & Canada)

Fax number: 314-447-8029

Elsevier Health Sciences Division
Subscription Customer Service
3251 Riverport Lane
Maryland Heights, MO 63043

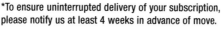

Printed and bound by CPI Group (UK) Ltd, Croydon, CR0 4YY

03/10/2024

01040359-0007